TAILORED
WEIGHT LOSS
Customizing Diets & Strategies for Different Body Types

Under no circumstances will the publisher or author be held liable for any damages, recovery, or financial loss due to the information contained in this book. Neither directly nor indirectly.

Legal Notice:
This book is protected by copyright. This book is for personal use only. You may not modify, distribute, sell, use, quote, or paraphrase any part or content of this book without the permission of the author or publisher.

Disclaimer Notice:
Please note that the information contained in this document is for educational and entertainment purposes only. Every effort has been made to present accurate, current, reliable, and complete information. No warranties of any kind are stated or implied. The reader acknowledges that the author is not offering legal, financial, medical, or professional advice. The contents of this book have been taken from various sources. Please consult a licensed professional before attempting any of the techniques described in this book.

By reading this document, the reader agrees that under no circumstances will the author be liable for any direct or indirect loss arising from the use of the information contained in this document, including but not limited to - errors, omissions, or inaccuracies.

INTRODUCTION

OVERVIEW OF WEIGHT LOSS CHALLENGES

You are beginning a journey that winds through the intricate landscape of weight reduction. It's a journey fraught with difficulties as different and singular as the people who travel it. Losing weight is a mosaic of mental struggles, emotional ups and downs, and social pressures in addition to physical challenges. Moving further, you will encounter an intimidating realm of contradictory data, where each turn of the corner reveals a fresh workout regimen or diet fad. "One-size-fits-all" is a prevalent phrase in this context. However, it is rarely accurate.

Your body is an individual, a special blueprint of demands and reactions. Thus, the struggle to lose weight becomes very personal. It's about knowing your body and how it works, hearing the whimpers and roars of its requirements, and adjusting your strategy appropriately. In "Tailored Weight Loss," you will discover that an ectomorphic frame that finds it difficult to maintain weight needs a different approach than a mesomorphic body that easily gains muscle. A different method is also necessary for the endomorphic body due to its inclination to accumulate fat.

Remind yourself as you turn each page that this is about gaining knowledge, not just losing weight. You'll have the ability to see past trends and identify what actually works for you. With the help of this book, you should be able to find a weight loss plan that honors your uniqueness amidst the chaos. It's an agreement to help you discover the language of your body and to carve out a unique path that is all your own. This is the core idea behind

"Tailored Weight Loss"—a personalized and self-exploration journey towards a healthier you.

UNDERSTANDING BODY TYPES

Before you start this trip, it's important to understand that every person's body is distinct, just like every fingerprint, with its own set of traits and preferences. Because every body type, whether endomorph, mesomorph, or ectomorph, reacts differently to diet and exercise, there is no one-size-fits-all answer. Knowing your body type involves more than scientific classification; it involves removing the layers to uncover the unique story of your metabolism, muscular makeup, and fat distribution.

As you peruse "Tailored Weight Loss," you'll discover that an ectomorph, who is long and slender, may find it difficult to put on weight and muscle, necessitating a diet high in calories to tip the scales. The mesomorph, who is naturally well-built and strong, may have an easier time controlling their weight, but they still need to be careful to keep their balance. Then there is the endomorph, which is often rounder and more likely to accumulate fat; in this case, diet and activity need to be properly balanced to tilt the scales in favor of losing weight.

However, these body kinds are only beginning points; they are not static groupings. They guide your dietary and activity choices, but they don't control your destiny. Your body is flexible, changeable, and responsive to the proper types of exercise and nourishment. You will discover how to take advantage of your body type and tailor your weight loss program to your unique physiological terrain in the upcoming chapters. "Tailored Weight Loss" is your manual for comprehending these body types and utilizing that information to design a weight loss plan that is unique to you.

THE IMPORTANCE OF PERSONALIZED WEIGHT LOSS APPROACHES

Personalized weight loss methods are not an extravagance; they are essential. Even though your DNA is unique, your route to losing weight and being healthy cannot be exactly the same as someone else's. "Tailored Weight Loss" is based on the idea that a customized approach that complements your body's unique demands and rhythms holds the key to long-term weight loss, rather than general diets or prefabricated exercise regimens.

You'll discover, as you read through the core of this book, that one-size-fits-all diets are frequently difficult and unsuccessful, like trying to fit square pegs into round holes. Your lifestyle, hormonal balance, metabolic rate, and sleep habits significantly affect your weight. It's critical to comprehend these aspects of your health because they have a direct impact on how well your weight loss attempts go.

This book will help you create a weight loss strategy as individual as your fingerprints. It will help you pay attention to the cues your body sends you, decipher what it requires, and react with decisions that best suit your needs. "Tailored Weight Loss" can assist you in piecing together the components of your weight reduction journey, whether it's the foods that fuel you most efficiently, the kinds of exercise that work best for you, or the lifestyle adjustments that have the biggest effects.

Here, you will discover how to respect the unique qualities of your body by using a weight loss strategy that acknowledges and honors it. The outcome? A happier, healthier version of yourself who understands that individualized weight loss plans that are both thoughtful and practical are the path to success rather than one built on restriction.

PART I: UNDERSTANDING BODY TYPES AND WEIGHT LOSS

CHAPTER 1: THE SCIENCE OF BODY TYPES

Knowing your body type is like learning your metabolism's language when losing weight. Start a conversation about changing your relationship with your body. Psychologist William Sheldon first suggested the idea of body types, or somatotypes, in the 1940s. He proposed three main types of body compositions: ectomorphic, mesomorphic, and endomorphic. This theory has been improved upon today, and although only some fall neatly into these categories, they offer a useful basis for customizing your weight loss strategy.

Ectomorphs are usually described as having a long, lean body type. An ectomorph's rapid metabolism can make it difficult to develop fat and muscle. Although this may appear advantageous, it can have drawbacks if you want to increase muscle mass or definition. Your weight loss strategy may focus more on developing lean muscle mass through resistance exercise and nutrient-rich diets than on dropping pounds.

Mesomorphs typically have a naturally athletic physique with distinct muscle groups. This body type may make it simpler for you to acquire muscle and control your weight. On the other hand, if you eat more calories than you expend, complacency might result in weight gain. Mesomorphs benefit from a balanced diet and an exercise regimen that combines cardio and strength training.

Endomorphs typically have greater body fat percentages and a propensity to accumulate fat, especially in the lower body. Although difficult, losing weight can still be achieved by endomorphs with a sluggish metabolism. To achieve a calorie deficit—which is necessary for weight loss—a low-carb diet and frequent aerobic exercise can be helpful.

However, how does science explain these different body types? Your hormonal balance and metabolic rate are influenced by your somatotype. For example, endomorphs with higher amounts of the hormone leptin may become less sensitive to satiety cues, which may result in overeating. Ectomorphs have a faster metabolism because, in general, the thyroid hormone, which controls metabolism, is more active in them.

Where you store fat also depends on your body type. Visceral fat, the harmful kind that envelops organs, is rarely accumulated by ectomorphs. Different body types have different tendencies regarding fat accumulation and loss. Mesomorphs are more prone to visceral fat build-up, but they can also effectively reduce it through exercise and a healthy diet. On the other hand, endomorphs tend to accumulate subcutaneous fat around their hips and thighs, which is less harmful than visceral fat but more challenging to get rid of.

This knowledge of body types is useful in real-world situations and is not only academic. It can help you identify more successful tactics and explain why you have previously failed with various diets. It can also clarify why you don't see effects from some activities while others do. This tool helps you sort through the clutter of weight reduction advice and identify a plan that aligns with your body's natural tendencies.

Remember that body types are easy and fast as you read on. People tend to be mixed kinds, and physical characteristics can alter over time. Numerous factors, including age, way of life, hormone levels, and others, might impact one's somatotype. Rather than placing you in a certain group, "Tailored Weight Loss" aims to give you a foundation for comprehending and interacting with your body.

In the upcoming chapters, we'll look at how to identify your body type, how genetics and environment shape it, and how to utilize this information to create a weight loss strategy that feels customized for you. Now is the time to translate the understanding of body types into a workable weight loss plan. Welcome to a fresh perspective on the state of your body and well-being.

DEFINITION AND CLASSIFICATION OF BODY TYPES

Body type classification and understanding are fundamental to health and fitness, especially when customizing training and weight loss regimens. It's the scientific understanding that all bodies are different and that each one needs a customized strategy to meet individual health objectives. The complex world of somatotypes is explored in this chapter, which also offers a road map for navigating the territory of individual physicality.

William Herbert Sheldon, a psychologist, created the idea of somatotypes in the early 1900s. Ectomorphs, mesomorphs, and endomorphs were the three main body forms he suggested for all human bodies. This trio provides a foundation for comprehending predispositions and body composition, providing a framework for creating individualized exercise and nutrition regimens.

Typically, ectomorphs have a tiny bone structure, a low body fat percentage, and a slender, linear appearance. Characterized by a rapid metabolism, this type finds it difficult to gain weight, both in muscle and fat. For an ectomorph to gain muscle, their diet may need to be higher in calories and incorporate more weight exercise.

Mesomorphs are in the middle of the somatotype continuum; they have medium-sized bones and well-defined muscles, and they are frequently naturally athletic. Their propensity to grow muscle and burn fat relatively easily gives them a major fitness advantage. The finest results are usually obtained by mesomorphs with a well-rounded diet and a balanced approach to strength and cardio exercise.

Endomorphs frequently have larger bone structures along with more body fat and total mass. Because of their slower metabolism, this kind may find it more difficult to lose weight. To increase metabolism and encourage fat loss, endomorphs frequently employ higher-intensity training and a restricted diet.

It's crucial to remember that only some fit neatly into one group, even while Sheldon's classifications offer a useful place to start. Most people display a variety of traits, which has led to the creation of terminology that describes these combinations, such as meso-endomorph and ecto-mesomorph. To create the best diet and exercise regimens, you must determine where you are on this spectrum.

Understanding the hormonal and metabolic variations that each type may display adds to the intricacy of body typing. For example, the thyroid hormone concentrations in ectomorphs are frequently higher, which can speed up metabolism. Endomorphs may be more likely to develop insulin resistance, which means they need to watch how many carbohydrates they eat.

Beyond characteristics of the body and metabolic predispositions, the classification takes into account the way the body reacts to various forms of exercise and nutrition. Ectomorphs, for instance, would benefit more from longer cardio workouts to maximize calorie burn, whereas endomorphs might benefit more from shorter, more intense bursts of activity to prevent catabolism (muscle loss).

Understanding that somatotypes are dynamic is also crucial. Your body type can be influenced by environmental influences, changes in lifestyle, and training adaptations. Just as an endomorph may shed fat and define their muscles with regular exercise and dietary control, so too can an ectomorph achieve noticeable muscular growth via focused strength training and nutrition.

Several procedures, including physical examinations, body composition analyses, and introspection about past struggles and achievements with weight control, may be used to identify your body type. You will learn how to determine your somatotype, comprehend its ramifications, and put this information to use in real-world situations with the help of this chapter.

Equipped with the knowledge gained from this chapter, you can proceed with a more comprehensive comprehension of your physical self. With this knowledge, you may work with your genetic predispositions to reach your fitness and weight loss goals rather than being condemned to a certain fate.

GENETIC AND ENVIRONMENTAL INFLUENCES ON BODY TYPE

Every person's body type is a unique pattern created by the interweaving of genetic and environmental forces. Although the categorization of body kinds offers a structure, the combination of genetics and environment customizes this structure for each individual. This interaction affects not just our physical makeup but also how our bodies react to certain lifestyle elements like exercise and nutrition.

Our bodies' potential is mapped out by our genetics, which also determines our height, bone structure, muscle fiber composition, and fat distribution. Our predisposition to be an ectomorph, mesomorph, or endomorph is determined by these genetic variables. For example, some people are genetically inclined to be more ectomorphic due to a higher metabolism, whereas other people may have genes that promote fat storage, which indicates an endomorphic propensity.

However, genes are not the only designers of our bodies. Our body types can be substantially altered by environmental circumstances, varying from stress levels and sleep habits to nutrition and physical activity. For instance, a regular resistance training regimen and a high-calorie diet may cause an ectomorph's physique to become more mesomorphic. On the other hand, a sedentary lifestyle and excess calories can give endomorphic traits to a mesomorph.

How our bodies respond to exercise is another example of how heredity and environment interact. Our muscle fiber type preponderance can be influenced by genetic variables, which can also affect our suitability for explosive power movements or endurance activities. Training can, however, cause a certain amount of muscle fiber-type transformation, demonstrating the body's amazing capacity to adjust to environmental demands.

Nutrition fulfills a similar dual function. Our dietary choices and eating habits also have a significant impact on our metabolism, even though genetics can also affect our metabolic rate and the way our bodies digest different macronutrients. To maximize metabolic health, a diet customized to a person's genetic makeup must be flexible enough to accommodate lifestyle modifications and age-related metabolic changes.

Furthermore, the environment we are raised in can have a long-lasting impact on the composition of our bodies. Regardless of genetic predispositions, a person reared in a diet-rich environment without encouragement for physical activity may acquire a body type that reflects these settings. On the other hand, distinct components of one's genetic potential may manifest in an individual who has access to a healthy diet and leads an active lifestyle.

As the twenty-first century progresses, epigenetics—the study of how our actions and surroundings can alter our genes—becomes increasingly important. We now know that specific environmental exposures can switch genes on or off, influencing a person's somatotype all their lives. This dynamic perspective on genetics and environment highlights that we actively shape our bodies rather than being passive recipients of our DNA.

Comprehending these factors is essential while creating a training or weight-management regimen. It necessitates a customized strategy that adapts to one's changing surroundings and way of life. For example, a person may need to modify their weight management strategy if they experience a change in their lifestyle, such as pregnancy, menopause, or new work with greater physical demands.

This chapter shows how our life experiences and inherent qualities interact in a complex dance that shapes our body types. By recognizing the roles played by genetics and environment, we may work together to design more adaptive and successful weight- and health-management solutions, bridging the gap between nature and nurture.

CHAPTER 2: METABOLISM AND BODY TYPES

Understanding Metabolism

The word "metabolism" comes up frequently while discussing exercise and weight loss. Food is transformed into energy by a biochemical process that is a continuous and essential aspect of life. Your body's total chemical reactions keep your cells alive and operating, and consequently, you make up your metabolism, which is more than just how rapidly you burn calories.

The first step in comprehending metabolism is to differentiate between the essential processes, anabolism and catabolism. Anabolism refers to the process of synthesizing various chemicals that are required by the cells, whereas catabolism involves breaking down molecules to obtain energy. Together, they form the fundamental energy cycle in your body, representing the yin and yang of chemical reactions.

Your basal metabolic rate (BMR) is the speed at which your body carries out these metabolic functions. These calories your body needs to function normally at rest, such as breathing and blood circulation. Your BMR can be affected by multiple factors, including genetics, age, sex, and body size. People with more muscular mass usually have a higher BMR because, for example, muscle burns more calories at rest than fat does.

Your metabolism might also be affected by your somatotype. Ectomorphs may have higher BMRs because of greater heat loss due to their high surface area-to-volume ratio. Compared to endomorphs, who may have a lower BMR because of a higher proportion of fat tissue, mesomorphs often have a higher BMR because of their greater muscle mass.

However, lifestyle choices can impact metabolism, which is not a static characteristic. For example, increasing muscle mass through physical exercise increases metabolic rate, increasing calorie burning even during rest. The diet also has an impact; specific meals and eating habits can speed up or slow down your metabolism momentarily.

Another part of metabolism is thermogenesis, which is the body's heat production process. It comprises both the energy utilized during physical activity and the energy required for food digestion, often called the thermic effect of food (TEF). The body uses energy to produce heat during even the simplest acts of thermogenesis, such as shivering in the cold.

Understanding metabolic adaptability is essential to comprehending weight loss. Your body adjusts to lower calorie intake by slowing down the rate at which it uses energy. This is why weight reduction can eventually plateau and why it's crucial to maintain your metabolism by combining nutrition and exercise.

Your body type and metabolism interact in a complicated way. Your somatotype doesn't determine your metabolic fate, even though it can provide you some insight into your innate metabolic tendencies. By adopting certain lifestyle choices, such as using strength training to gain muscle mass or high-intensity interval training (HIIT) to increase your metabolic rate after exercise, you can increase your metabolism.

Developing an efficient weight loss plan requires an understanding of metabolism about body types. For ectomorphs, maintaining a naturally high metabolic rate may need a diet high in calories. Mesomorphs might gain from a well-rounded strategy that uses their ability to gain muscle to keep their metabolism strong. Endomorphs may concentrate on strength training and frequent cardio activity to increase their metabolic rate.

You'll learn about the complexities of metabolism and how to work with your body, not against it, to reach your health and weight loss objectives as this chapter progresses. Understanding metabolism will help you on your path to becoming a healthier version of yourself by enabling you to customize your diet and exercise regimen to fit your own metabolic blueprint.

HOW DIFFERENT BODY TYPES AFFECT METABOLISM

One important aspect of the weight loss puzzle is understanding the relationship between metabolism and body types. Your somatotype is one of the many elements that affect your metabolism, the bodily engine that powers your daily activities and burns calories. To provide you with the information to take advantage of your unique metabolic quirks, this chapter will examine how each body type interacts with and influences metabolic processes.

Ectomorphs typically have a high metabolism and are distinguished by their tall, lean, and frequently delicate frames. Ectomorphs typically struggle with gaining weight rather than reducing it. Ectomorphs can consume more calories without necessarily experiencing noticeable changes in weight because of their rapid metabolic rate. Higher sympathetic nervous system activity, which frequently results in increased calorie burn, is the cause of this quick metabolism. To build muscle, ectomorphs may need a specialized strength-training program and a diet rich in protein and carbohydrates.

Because of their naturally muscular and athletic frame, mesomorphs usually have better-balanced metabolisms. This body type's metabolism is sensitive to changes in food and activity, allowing it to grow muscle and lose fat easily. To preserve their muscular tone and metabolic balance, mesomorphs gain from a varied training regimen incorporating strength and cardio activities.

In contrast, endomorphs are typically rounder and stockier, and they typically have a lower metabolic rate. Because endomorphs may acquire weight more easily and lose it more difficult, this can make weight management more difficult. A slower metabolism indicates that the body stores foods as fat more effectively than burns for energy. Endomorphs can jump-start their slow metabolism and encourage fat reduction by combining frequent cardio and metabolic training with a protein-rich, low-carb diet.

The ratio of muscle to fat helps explain some of the variation in metabolic rates among the various body types. Because muscle tissue has an active metabolism, even while at rest, it needs more energy to be maintained. As a result, compared to endomorphs, mesomorphs, and muscular ectomorphs typically have higher resting metabolic rates. On the other hand, as many endomorphs have more adipose (fat) tissue than muscle, this type of tissue is less metabolically active than muscle and can lead to a lower total metabolic rate.

Nevertheless, body type is not the only factor that affects metabolism. Age, gender, hormonal balances, and lifestyle decisions all matter. For example, thyroid hormones play a major role in controlling metabolic rate, and changes in these hormones can significantly affect how quickly or slowly your body burns calories.

Furthermore, it's important to understand the idea of metabolic flexibility, or the body's capacity to quickly switch between burning fats and carbs for energy. Mesomorphs frequently exhibit high levels of metabolic adaptability, which can be useful for preserving body composition. Because they require more energy, ectomorphs may tend to burn more carbohydrates, but endomorphs may need more effort to develop their metabolic flexibility to effectively manage their weight.

You will go deeper into the tactics that affect and even improve your metabolism in this chapter. Creating a diet and fitness program that suits you requires an understanding of the metabolic preferences of your particular body type. It's about establishing a balanced relationship between your food intake, your physical activity level, and your body's energy utilization so that you can effectively and sustainably lose weight.

METABOLIC RATE AND WEIGHT LOSS

The rate at which your body uses up energy or burns calories is known as your metabolic rate, and it is a key factor in weight loss. It establishes your basal metabolic rate, or the minimum calories required to sustain your body's essential processes (BMR). About 60–75% of your total energy expenditure is accounted for by your BMR; the remaining portion is required for physical activity and the thermic effect of food (TEF)—the process of breaking down food.

You need to consume fewer calories than your body expels to lose weight. Therefore, a key determinant in deciding how quickly or slowly you lose weight is the pace of your metabolism. While a lower metabolic rate can have the opposite effect, a greater metabolic rate can result in speedier energy expenditure and simpler weight reduction.

The following variables affect your metabolic rate: body size, muscular mass, age, sex, and heredity. In general, men's metabolic rates are higher than women's and decline with age. Your metabolic rate will increase with muscle mass because muscular tissue has a higher metabolic activity than fat tissue. For this reason, increasing muscle mass and strength training are frequently advised to speed up metabolism.

Understanding metabolic rate and weight reduction also requires an understanding of energy balance. The link between the energy you consume (calories from food and drink) and the energy you expend (calories expended via physical activity and fundamental body functions) is known as energy balance. Your weight won't change if your intake and expenditure are in balance. You will lose weight if your intake is less than your expenditure.

A further component of metabolism that influences weight loss is adaptive thermogenesis. It describes how the body modifies its basal metabolic rate (BMR) in response to variations in energy intake or expenditure. For instance, your body may adjust by slowing down your metabolism to conserve energy when you drastically reduce your calorie intake, making it more difficult to lose weight over time.

The aspect that you have the most control over in terms of your overall energy expenditure is physical activity. Running and cycling are aerobic exercises that temporarily boost your energy expenditure. On the other hand, over time, gaining muscle raises your energy expenditure since, even at rest, muscle burns more calories than fat.

Hormones also have a big impact on weight loss and metabolic rate. Your metabolism can be sped up or slowed down by imbalances in thyroid hormones, which control your body mass index. Another hormone that influences how your body stores and uses energy, particularly glucose, is insulin.

A common mistake made by people trying to lose weight is to drastically cut their calorie intake. This can result in a significant decrease in metabolic rate and cause a plateau in weight loss. This can be lessened by increasing physical activity, particularly muscle-strengthening activities to increase lean body mass and boost metabolic rate, and implementing a progressive, moderate calorie deficit.

Comprehending your basal metabolic rate is crucial for successful weight reduction. It is a variable that can be impacted by lifestyle decisions rather than a fixed quantity. To maximize your total energy expenditure, a successful weight loss plan includes physical activity and dieting. You can customize your weight-reduction plan to match your metabolic rate by learning how your body burns energy. This will help you reach and sustain your weight loss objectives over time.

CHAPTER 3: PSYCHOLOGICAL ASPECTS OF BODY TYPES

Body Image and Self-Esteem

Self-esteem and body image are closely related, and they are quite individualized. Your perception of your body has a big influence on how you feel about yourself and how you move around the environment. This chapter delves into the psychological fabric that entwines self-esteem and body image, especially about body kinds.

The mental or subjective representation of one's own body is called body image. It's your internal representation, which might or might not be true. Contrarily, self-esteem is the total feeling of one's value or worth. Individual experiences, cultural influences, and internalized standards all impact both.

Every bodily type—ectomorph, mesomorph, or endomorph—is associated with stigmas and preconceptions from society that can affect how each person views. Being viewed as weak or flimsy, ectomorphs may experience pressure to become voluptuous or more muscular. Mesomorphs, often valued for their athletic build, may experience pressure to uphold a particular physical appearance to conform to social norms. Endomorphs frequently fight against the stigma of obesity and the presumption of bad habits, even though they may have trouble controlling their weight.

These preconceptions have the potential to cause negative self-evaluation and a skewed body image, which can lower self-esteem. For example, internalizing negative body image stereotypes can make someone feel insecure, which can affect how they interact with others and make personal decisions. This can lead to a situation known as a "self-fulfilling prophecy," in which the person's actions support their poor self-esteem and reinforce their negative self-image.

The media can intensify feelings of inadequacy and have a significant influence on how people feel about their bodies. Unrealistic standards for physical beauty can be brought about by constant exposure to photos of "ideal" bodies that are either unachievable or digitally changed. The difference between a person's perception of their physique and the "ideal" can damage self-worth, which can result in negative behaviors like binge eating disorders or excessive exercise.

However, the relationship between self-esteem and body image is not one-way; raising one's self-esteem can produce a more positive perception of one's physique. No matter what form or size your body is, you're more likely to recognize its unique qualities and skills when you value who you are and your inherent worth.

It's important to tackle changes regarding body types and weight loss with self-compassion and an awareness that worth and health are not exclusively based on outward looks. It is crucial to adopt a comprehensive perspective on health that takes mental and emotional well-being into account. Establishing attainable, health-oriented objectives instead of purely aesthetic ones can promote a good body image and increase self-worth.

Creating a welcoming atmosphere is also essential. A healthy body image can be strengthened by being in communities that support body acceptance and surrounding yourself with good influences. Meditation and gratitude journaling are two examples of mindfulness exercises that can assist in changing attention from outward appearances to resilience and inner attributes.

Understanding that your body type is just one part of who you are can enable you to value your body's functionality as much as its appearance. Instead of obsessing about the number on the scale, celebrate your little accomplishments, like increased strength or endurance, since these can boost your self-confidence and foster a more positive relationship with your body.

We'll discuss body image and self-esteem-building techniques, body type-related psychological obstacles, and how a good self-perception can support long-term, healthful living. It's a transformative journey where you learn to understand and confidently embrace your individuality while navigating the psychological terrain of body types.

EMOTIONAL EATING AND STRESS MANAGEMENT

Emotional eating is a prevalent stress-reduction strategy in which food is consumed to numb or repress unpleasant feelings. This kind of eating is motivated by emotions rather than hunger. Food becomes an emotional salve, a transient escape from the complexity of life, whether it is from sadness, anxiety, boredom, or delight.

Life will always involve stress, which has a significant effect on eating patterns and weight control. The hormone cortisol, released by the body in response to stress, can enhance hunger and desires for foods heavy in fat and sugar. These "comfort foods" activate the brain's reward regions, which produce a brief feeling of relaxation and pleasure. This temporary solace is frequently followed by emotions of guilt and shame, which can feed the vicious cycle of emotional eating.

To control emotional eating, it is crucial to identify the reasons behind it. Being aware of the underlying causes is the first step towards managing this behavior effectively. It necessitates introspection and awareness of the emotional factors that trigger food desires. Workplace stress, marital problems, money worries, health concerns, and even exhaustion are common causes. Finding these triggers enables the creation of non-food coping mechanisms as an alternative.

Mindfulness is a useful tactic for controlling stress and emotional eating. You can increase your awareness of your eating patterns and the emotions that influence them by engaging in mindfulness practices. By slowing down the eating process, methods like mindful eating—which centers on the eating experience—can improve the perception of hunger and fullness cues.

Developing a toolset of stress-reduction strategies is another essential part of controlling emotional eating. Because regular exercise releases endorphins, it is a stress relief and mood enhancer. Engaging in enjoyable activities, like yoga, dancing, or brisk walks, might offer a healthy way to decompress.

Other effective stress-reducing techniques include progressive muscle relaxation, deep breathing exercises, and meditation. They can lessen the need to turn to food for emotional solace, relax the mind, and lower cortisol levels. Developing a routine can help you feel in control and at ease, which lowers the chance of emotional eating.

To control stress and emotional eating, social support is essential. Talking to loved ones, friends, or a support group about your worries might help you feel better and gain perspective. Sometimes, expressing your emotions might lessen their influence and curb your desire to eat.

Additionally, journaling can be a therapeutic technique by facilitating the private, introspective expression of feelings. Writing down your thoughts and feelings might make it easier to spot emotional eating patterns and encourage the creation of more positive coping mechanisms for stressful situations.

Some people have strong emotional eating habits and can benefit from expert assistance. Cognitive-behavioral therapy (CBT) can help people create new, healthier coping skills and alter the mental processes that cause emotional eating.

Regular, well-balanced meals and snacks help control blood sugar levels and ward off severe hunger, which can lead to emotional eating. Having wholesome snacks and meal planning will help lessen the chance of stress-induced impulsive eating.

Stress-reduction strategies, social support, professional counseling, and mindfulness are all effective ways to control emotional eating as a reaction to stress. It is possible to stop the cycle of emotional eating and create a better connection with food by identifying the emotional triggers and creating a thorough stress management plan.

SETTING REALISTIC GOALS

Any successful venture starts with setting realistic goals, but it's crucial to managing weight and health. Achievable and quantifiable, realistic goals give your efforts a clear direction. They also support the sustenance of motivation and a sense of achievement that will aid you in the long run.

Recognizing your current situation and desired future state is the first step toward creating realistic goals. This calls for an open evaluation of your lifestyle, skills, and state of health. It's critical to accept where you are as a beginner without passing judgment and to understand that improvement is a methodical process that takes tiny, incremental steps.

Specifying your goals is crucial while defining them. Ambitious goals such as "I want to lose weight" or "I want to be healthier" are not specific enough to direct your efforts. A particular objective would be, "I aim to lose 10 pounds in 10 weeks by incorporating a balanced diet and regular exercise into my routine." This precision helps you plan the essential actions to get there and provides you with a precise target to shoot for.

Measurable objectives must also be realistic. You may monitor your progress and make any adjustments by putting your goals into numerical form. The issues of how much, how many, and how I will know when the goal has been met are all addressed by measurable goals.

Realistic goal-setting also requires realistic goals to be attainable. Your goals should challenge you but be manageable. You will only end up frustrated and disappointed if you set an unrealistically high target. Instead, pick a goal that will require work and attention but is still doable.

Realistic goal-setting also requires relevance. Your objectives must align with your beliefs, passions, and stage of life. They should be significant to you individually, not determined by what you should do in the eyes of others. Objectives have greater meaning and are more inspiring when they are pertinent.

Time-bound objectives provide you a deadline to help you prioritize and maintain focus. You may be inspired to take action by the sense of urgency it instills. A time-bound objective, such as "I will increase my daily step count to 10,000 steps within the next 30 days," provides you with a specific deadline for completion.

It's crucial to think about potential obstacles and plan how you'll overcome them while making goals. You can plan strategies by anticipating issues, which increases your likelihood of staying on course when they do.

Establishing goals requires flexibility as well. Because life is unpredictable, things might change suddenly. Be ready to review your objectives and make any necessary adjustments. Adaptability lets you deal with changes while maintaining sight of your ultimate goals.

It's essential to acknowledge little accomplishments along the road to stay motivated. No matter how tiny, acknowledge each step you take in the correct path. This keeps you involved in the process and reinforces great conduct.

Finally, keep in mind to be gentle with yourself. Progress is frequently non-linear and requires time to manifest. Ups and downs are inevitable, but the important thing is to persevere and never waver from your objectives.

Specificity, measurability, achievability, relevancy, and time-bound criteria are all necessary for setting realistic goals. It also calls for patience, adaptability, anticipating obstacles, and acknowledging advancements. By establishing reasonable objectives, you build a successful plan that may result in long-term transformation and enhanced well-being.

PART II: DIET AND NUTRITION STRATEGIES FOR EACH BODY TYPE

CHAPTER 4: DIET FOR ECTOMORPHS

The slim physique, rapid metabolism, and inability to put on weight or muscle mass are common characteristics of ectomorphs. For an ectomorph, the goal of a healthy diet is to consume more calories to support energy requirements and muscle building. You will be guided through creating an ectomorphic body type-appropriate diet in this chapter.

First and foremost, ectomorphs must consume more calories than they expend. You should aim for three big meals and two to three substantial snacks throughout the day because of your fast metabolism. Maintaining consistency is essential, as sporadic meals may result in inadequate calorie intake to meet your energy requirements.

Ectomorphs should prioritize a larger amount of carbs when it comes to macronutrients. Good carbs give you the energy you need to power your rapid metabolism. Examples of these include whole grains, fruits, and vegetables. This means that carbohydrates should make up 50-60% of the total calories you consume. Low-GI complex carbohydrates offer a consistent release of energy, making them the better option.

For muscles to grow and heal, protein is also necessary. Aim for a moderate protein intake of 25–30% calories as an ectomorph. Fish, eggs, dairy products, legumes, nuts, and lean meats are good protein sources. You can ensure that you get enough protein by including a source of protein in each meal and snack.

Since they are high in calories and can aid in achieving your calorie target, fats should be considered. Fats, especially unsaturated fats in avocados, nuts, seeds, and olive oil, should comprise about 20–25% of your daily caloric intake. Not only are these fats beneficial to general health, but they also help produce hormones, which are essential for building muscle.

Drinking enough water is also crucial, particularly if you exercise frequently. Both general health and muscle function must drink lots of water throughout the day.

Regarding supplements, ectomorphs may find that muscle gainers or protein powders help you consume more protein and calories. It's crucial to remember that supplements are exactly that—a supplement to a diet already rich in nutrients.

Lastly, one way to maximize your nutrition is through meal scheduling. Before and after your workouts, eating a meal or snack high in protein and carbohydrates can help support the growth and recuperation of your muscles.

For the ectomorph diet to support muscle growth and an active lifestyle, it should be high in calories, rich in high-quality carbohydrates, and contain enough protein and healthy fats. An effective dietary plan for ectomorphs includes regular, well-balanced meals and snacks, adequate water, and thoughtful meal timing. Ectomorphs can conquer their innate inclination toward leanness and attain their ideal body and health objectives with the appropriate eating plan.

CHARACTERISTICS OF ECTOMORPHS

Ectomorphs are one of the three body compositions, or somatotypes, frequently used to characterize an individual's morphology. They are easily recognized by their slender, linear build and quick metabolism, a distinguishing characteristic that influences their capacity to put on weight and muscle. Comprehending the attributes of ectomorphs is vital in customizing diet and exercise regimens to suit their unique requirements.

Ectomorphs often have small bone structures, narrow shoulders and chests, and slender limbs. They are also typically tall and thin. Their body's tendency to burn off extra calories due to a high basal metabolic rate (BMR) is often the cause of their slim build. This implies that ectomorphs, typically coveted by people more concerned about their weight, can consume large amounts of food without gaining weight.

Ectomorphs frequently struggle to put on muscle mass. The fast-twitch muscle fibers that give rise to the growth and strength acquired through resistance training are often less prevalent in them. Rather, their muscles might be better adapted to endurance, making them inherently better at sports like cycling or long-distance running.

Ectomorphs have a faster metabolism and higher energy consumption due to their dominance of the sympathetic nervous system in their metabolism. This might help keep a trim figure, but it can also be difficult for people who want to gain or increase muscle.

Ectomorphs' lightweight frames and quick metabolism allow them to succeed in endurance and agility-based exercise activities. Ectomorphs may need to participate in a more focused and rigorous strength training regimen, frequently accompanied by a greater caloric intake to support muscle growth and recovery to increase strength and muscle mass.

Ectomorphs usually need a higher dietary intake of carbohydrates to maintain their energy levels. To satisfy their body's needs, they frequently need to eat more regularly and ensure they get enough calories. To supply enough vitamins and minerals to support an active lifestyle and metabolic needs, their meals should be centered on foods high in nutrients.

Additionally, ectomorphs typically have a higher tolerance for carbohydrates, and they react better to carb loading, which is advantageous for endurance-based exercises. To maintain general health and muscle anabolism, they must still balance their macronutrient consumption with sufficient amounts of fat and protein.

Psychologically, ectomorphs' perceptions of their bodies can be shaped by individual objectives and societal norms. Ectomorphs may experience pressure to put on weight and muscle to conform to social norms that equate femininity with curves or strength and masculinity despite the idealization of their slender shape in fashion.

Knowing what ectomorphs are like will help you create exercise, nutrition, and health plans that work for you. Understanding the benefits and drawbacks of this body type can help ectomorphs make the most of their diet and exercise regimens to reach their unique objectives for body composition and overall health.

MACRONUTRIENT RATIOS AND CALORIC INTAKE

A balanced diet must include both macronutrient ratios and calorie consumption. These are crucial for reaching various fitness and health objectives, such as weight loss, muscle gain, and general well-being. The body uses macronutrients —carbohydrates, proteins, and fats—as its three main energy sources, and each one is essential to various body processes.

The body uses mostly carbohydrates as fuel, especially when performing high-intensity activity and powering the brain. Muscle is composed of proteins, which are necessary for both growth and repair. Fats are essential for hormone synthesis, nutrient absorption, and energy provision, especially during low-intensity exercise. The ideal macronutrient ratio varies based on personal goals, exercise level, and metabolic health.

The Institute of Medicine's Acceptable Macronutrient Distribution Ranges (AMDR) recommend the following distribution for weight control and overall health:
45–65% of calories come from carbs.
- Protein accounts for 10–35% of calories.
Amount of fat in calories: 20–35%

Those who want to lose weight can change these ratios to include more protein, which can improve satiety and help maintain muscle mass during a calorie deficit. Reducing carbohydrate consumption may also be advantageous for people on a ketogenic diet or those who have insulin resistance. To sustain lengthy activities, endurance athletes might need more calories from carbohydrates.

Suppose an ectomorph or bodybuilder is having trouble gaining mass. In that case, the macronutrient ratio may change to - 50–60% of calories from carbohydrates to gain muscle.
- Protein accounts for 25–30% of calories.
Amount of fat in calories (20–30%)

This change guarantees enough protein for muscle synthesis and repair, enough glycogen stores for hard training, and healthy fats for hormonal balance and recuperation.

Macronutrient ratios are important, but so is calorie consumption. A person has to consume calories equal to their total daily energy expenditure (TDEE) to maintain their weight. While weight gain demands a calorie surplus, weight loss requires a caloric deficit—consuming fewer calories than the TDEE. It's crucial to remember that extreme calorie surpluses or deficits may have unfavorable effects.

Finding the BMR is the first step in calculating the appropriate calorie intake. This can be done using a variety of formulas, such as the Mifflin-St Jeor or Harris-Benedict formulas. After that, the TDEE is estimated by taking activity levels into account. Reducing daily intake by 500–1000 calories can safely lead to a weekly weight reduction of 1-2 pounds for a modest caloric deficit.

It's critical to adjust these ratios and calorie intake to meet the needs of each individual, taking into account variables like age, sex, height, weight, and metabolic health, as well as physical activity. To ensure that the diet stays in line with evolving goals and lifestyle circumstances, regular monitoring and modifications are made.

The key to reaching and sustaining ideal health results is a mindful approach to macronutrient ratios and calorie consumption, tailored to match individual goals and physiological needs.

SAMPLE MEAL PLANS AND FOODS

To achieve targeted health objectives, sample meal plans and foods that match certain dietary goals can be very helpful. Whether the goal is to maintain a balanced diet, develop muscle mass, or lose weight, following a planned meal plan with recommended foods will make things easier and guarantee that nutritional requirements are satisfied. This is a broad guide that can be adjusted based on personal calorie requirements and macronutrient ratios:

To Lose Weight:

Breakfast: - Egg whites, spinach, tomatoes, and mushrooms in an omelet
- Whole grain bread - A little portion of fresh fruit, such as an orange or berries

Snack: Greek yogurt drizzled with honey and chia seeds

Lunch consists of grilled chicken salad topped with cucumbers, cherry tomatoes, and mixed greens with a vinaigrette dressing.
- A portion of brown rice or quinoa

Snack: - Hummus with raw veggies like bell peppers and carrots

Supper will be baked salmon paired with sweet potatoes and steamed broccoli, along with a simple salad dressed with lemon juice.

To Gain Muscle:

Breakfast consists of scrambled eggs with avocado and diced bell peppers.
- Oatmeal topped with peanut butter and sliced bananas

Snack: A protein smoothie made with almond milk, whey protein, and a few oats

Lunch is a turkey breast sandwich with cheese, lettuce, and tomato on whole-grain bread.
- A baked potato wedge side dish

Snack: pieces of pineapple mixed with cottage cheese

Supper will be lentil soup and grilled steak paired with asparagus and quinoa salad.

With a Well-Balanced Diet:

Breakfast consists of sliced strawberries and whole grain cereal with almond milk and nuts.

Snack: Almond butter with apple slices

Lunch includes avocado, whole grain crackers, and tuna salad with mixed greens.

Snack: A tiny serving of dried fruit and mixed nuts

Dinner is miso soup and stir-fried tofu with a rainbow of bright vegetables over brown rice.

Foods You Should Eat:
Include a variety of foods in your diet that provide all the macronutrients for a well-balanced diet. Good sources of carbohydrates include whole grains such as quinoa, brown rice, and oats, starchy vegetables like sweet potatoes, and fiber-rich

fruits and vegetables. For lean proteins, consider foods such as fish, chicken, lentils, tofu, and dairy products like Greek yogurt. Avocados, almonds, seeds, olive oil, and fatty seafood like salmon are all good sources of healthy fats.

Recall that these meal plans are only examples and should be modified by personal dietary needs, preferences, and constraints. To fit your lifestyle and energy needs, it's also critical to consider portion sizes and meal scheduling. Getting advice from a nutritionist or dietitian might help you design a meal plan that suits your needs.

CHAPTER 5: DIET FOR MESOMORPHS

Typically, mesomorphs are distinguished by their innate strength, well-defined muscles, and naturally athletic frame. Compared to the other somatotypes, they have a modest frame and find it simpler to maintain a low body fat percentage and acquire muscle. Mesomorphs require specific food requirements to sustain muscular growth and maintain their active metabolism.

A balanced macronutrient distribution is essential for mesomorphs. The usual advice is to divide your intake into 40% fat, 30% protein, and 40% carbs. Using a balanced approach, mesomorphs can avoid unintended weight gain while having enough energy for exercises and muscle repair.

Complex carbs are key to a mesomorph's diet because they offer long-lasting energy and reduce insulin spikes. Starchy vegetables, legumes, and whole grains like quinoa, brown rice, and oats, as well as fruits and leafy greens, provide mesomorphs with adequate vitamins, minerals, and dietary fiber.

For mesomorphs to develop and repair muscular tissue, protein is essential. Regular mealtime inclusions should include high-quality protein sources, including fish, eggs, lean meats, and plant-based proteins like lentils, chickpeas, and tofu. Consuming protein in moderation throughout the day is recommended, particularly after exercise, to support muscle growth and repair.

Mesomorphs also require healthy lipids for hormone modulation, critical for both muscular growth and general health, in addition to their calorie density. Avocados, almonds, seeds, olive oil, and fatty fish high in omega-3 fatty acids are good sources of healthful fats.

Another important component of a mesomorph's diet is hydration. Consuming enough water helps the body's metabolism, muscles, and nutrient transportation. Because of their active lifestyle, mesomorphs need to drink plenty of water.

Mesomorphs may also gain by regulating their nutritional intake to maximize their recuperation and performance. Before and after exercise, eating a mix of carbohydrates and protein can improve muscle protein synthesis and restore glycogen levels.

This is an example of a mesomorph's daily menu:

Lunchtime:
- Almond butter and banana slices on top of oatmeal
Eggs scrambled or a protein shake

Peak:
- Tofu or grilled chicken breast - Mixed salad with colorful veggies and a drizzle of olive oil dressing
- Rice (brown or sweet)

Half:
- Sliced veggies with guacamole - Greek yogurt with mixed nuts

Supper:
- Quinoa or whole grain spaghetti - Steamed broccoli or asparagus
- Baked fish or lentil stew

Snack (if needed): A tiny serving of cottage cheese or a casein protein smoothie

Rich in nutrient-rich foods, the mesomorphic diet promotes muscle growth and an active lifestyle. Portion control is crucial because mesomorphs who consume more calories than they burn off may gain weight. Mesomorphs must follow a consistent diet and exercise schedule to preserve their muscular build and general well-being.

CHARACTERISTICS OF MESOMORPHS

Mesomorphs are regarded as the ideal athletic body type since they frequently possess a physique that many aspire to through diet and exercise. Their medium-sized frame, well-defined muscles, and effective metabolism that balance fat loss and muscle building distinguish them. Understanding mesomorph traits is crucial to maximizing their diet and exercise regimens to support their ideal body type and health objectives.

Physique and Muscle Composition: Mesomorphs usually have a rectangular-shaped body and an athletic, robust appearance. They have big shoulders, a narrow waist, and a broad chest. Mesomorphs have uniformly distributed muscle fibers throughout their bodies, which helps them look proportionate and balanced. Mesomorphs are naturally stronger and more powerful due to their increased proportion of fast-twitch muscle fibers; this makes them excellent at sports requiring quick bursts of strength and speed.

Metabolic Efficiency: Compared to other somatotypes, mesomorphs' bodies tend to burn calories more effectively, giving them a metabolic edge. When they adhere to a regular exercise schedule, they are more likely to maintain a favorable muscle-to-fat ratio, which makes it simpler to stay thin while still gaining muscle growth. Less frequently than endomorphs, mesomorphs can gain weight without regular exercise and a healthy diet, but their balanced metabolism makes it easier to shed extra pounds.

Exercise Response: Mesomorphs respond well to exercise, with noticeable and speedy results. They frequently see a noticeable increase in strength and fitness levels in a short amount of time and have tremendous potential for muscle growth. Because of their natural build and endurance, they may enjoy various physical activities and sports and frequently excel in them.

Dietary Considerations: Mesomorphs can have a rather varied diet due to their efficient metabolism, but they must still be aware of the balance between their macronutrients and calories. Although they have an efficient metabolism, they must combine their carbohydrate diet with high-quality proteins and healthy fats to maintain their energy levels and muscle mass.

Adaptability: The ability of the mesomorph's body to adjust to various training regimens is one of their greatest benefits. They make for a versatile and adaptable workout regimen because they can transition between strength and endurance training easily. Mesomorphs can customize their routines to meet certain objectives, such as fat loss, muscle building, or general fitness, thanks to their versatility.

Psychological Aspects: Mesomorphs could experience particular psychological difficulties. There may be an excessive focus on performance and appearance due to the strong social pressure to preserve one's "ideal" body type. Mesomorphs should prioritize exercise and health over appearance to promote a healthy body image and self-esteem.

Mesomorphs are usually muscular, athletic, and thin; they can put on muscle and maintain it reasonably easily. They are suitable for various physical activities due to their sensitive muscle fibers and effective metabolism. Mesomorphs can preserve their native body type and improve their health with a well-rounded workout program and a balanced diet.

BALANCING MACRONUTRIENTS FOR OPTIMAL PERFORMANCE

Whether they are athletes or fitness enthusiasts, balancing macronutrients—carbohydrates, proteins, and fats—is essential for optimizing physical performance. The body uses each macronutrient for a different purpose to function and supply energy. Having the proper balance of these nutrients will help you recover quickly after workouts and maintain better health overall.

Carbs: The Main Source of Energy

The body's primary energy source is carbs. They convert into glucose for immediate use or store as glycogen. Carbohydrates should make up a sizable amount of the diet for optimum performance, particularly during high-intensity or endurance sports. Usually, 45% to 65% of total calorie consumption is advised.

Whole grains, legumes, and starchy vegetables are complex carbs that offer a longer-lasting energy release. Simple carbs are also essential and can be found in fruits and dairy products. For rapid energy, however, they should be ingested closer to workout times.

Building and Repairing Muscle with Proteins

Muscle tissue growth, repair, and maintenance all depend on proteins. They are essential for muscular adaption, avoiding muscle deterioration, and recuperating from exercise. Protein requirements for individuals who train frequently can rise to 1.2 to 2.0 grams per kilogram of body weight per day, or 15% to 25% of total energy intake.

Lean meats, seafood, dairy products, eggs, and, for plant-based diets, lentils and soy products are good protein sources. Consuming protein in moderation throughout the day, particularly after exercise, can support muscle growth and repair.

Fats: A Source of Concentrated Energy

When glycogen is exhausted during prolonged exertion, the body switches to fat reserves, making fats a concentrated energy source. They are also necessary for the synthesis of hormones and the uptake of fat-soluble vitamins. Aim for 20% to 35% of calories from fats, primarily from unsaturated fats found in avocados, nuts, seeds, and fatty fish like salmon, which have anti-inflammatory properties and promote heart health in general.

Determining the Optimal Balance

Exercise types, length, intensity, and individual needs can all affect the ideal macronutrient balance. For instance, although strength athletes may place a higher priority on protein for muscle growth and repair, endurance athletes may need a higher intake of carbohydrates to sustain extended training sessions.

To be considered vitamins and hydration are also essential for peak performance. Maintaining blood volume and controlling body temperature requires enough fluid intake, while vitamins and minerals help with a wide range of biological processes, such as the creation of energy and the contraction of muscles.

To summarise, optimal athletic performance can be greatly

improved by maintaining a balanced intake of carbs, proteins, and fats based on individual requirements and training demands. To get the most out of consuming macronutrients, it's critical to modify these ratios when exercise routines vary and consider when to take nutrients.

SAMPLE MEAL PLANS AND FOODS

Achieving specific health goals and supplying the body with the necessary fuel for everyday activities requires the creation of sample meal plans that offer a balance of nutrients. The following sample meal plan provides a range of foods to satisfy the body's need for macronutrients throughout the day:

Breakfast: A Start to Boost Energy
- Cooked rolled oats with milk or a dairy-free substitute, combined with a dollop of protein powder, garnished with a spoonful of flaxseeds, fresh berries, and honey.
- For a dose of vitamin C, consume one orange whole or in the form of juice.

Mid-morning snack: Protein-Rich Pick-Me-Up – a slice of whole grain toast topped with avocado and cottage cheese or Greek yogurt with a sprinkling of granola and a handful of nuts.

Green tea increases antioxidant levels.

Lunch: satisfying and well-balanced
- A quinoa salad topped with diced tomatoes, cucumbers, and bell peppers, along with a side of mixed greens prepared with lemon juice and olive oil, accompanied by grilled chicken breast or chickpea patties.
. A fruit slice, like an apple or a pear, for a dessert high in fiber.

Snack in the Afternoon: Quick and Healthful
- Hummus paired with various raw veggies, such as bell pepper

slices, carrots, and celery.
- If you need a quick energy boost, eating a small portion of almonds and dried fruits can be very helpful.

Lunch: Full of Flavor and Nutrients
- Baked salmon or tofu steak served with steamed broccoli or asparagus and a side dish of sweet potato mash.
. a mixed green salad topped with sliced almonds, cherry tomatoes, and vinaigrette dressing.

Evening Snack: Comforting and Light
- A serving of mixed berries topped with whipped coconut cream or a casein protein smoothie.
- A cup of herbal tea to end the day.

Dishes to Incorporate: - Carbohydrates: Starchy vegetables (sweet potatoes, squash), fruits, legumes, whole grains (brown rice, quinoa, whole grain pasta, and oats).
Proteins: Fish (tuna, salmon), eggs, dairy products (cottage cheese, Greek yogurt), lean meats (turkey, chicken), and plant-based foods (lentils, tofu, and tempeh).
Fats: Avocados, fatty fish, nut butter, nuts and seeds, and olive oil.

The macronutrient balance in this meal plan is intended to maintain healthy energy levels, muscle regeneration, and general health. To make sure that micronutrient requirements are also satisfied, which is crucial for optimum body processes, it incorporates a range of dietary sources.

Remember that each person's dietary needs, tastes, and objectives should be considered when choosing portion sizes and particular foods. A dietitian consultation can offer individualized advice for designing meal plans that are suitable for you.

CHAPTER 6: DIET FOR ENDOMORPHS

Generally speaking, endomorphs have a fuller build, a greater body fat percentage, and a tendency to accumulate fat. They frequently have slower metabolisms, making controlling their weight more difficult. Nonetheless, endomorphs can successfully manage their weight and enhance their health using appropriate dietary techniques.

Endomorphs should emphasize increasing metabolism and decreasing fat storage in their diet. Here's an example of how endomorphs can arrange their food:

Ratios of Macronutrients:
A macronutrient ratio that prioritizes proteins and fats over carbohydrates—especially refined carbohydrates—may be advantageous for endomorphs. Reducing the amount of carbohydrates consumed can assist in controlling insulin levels, which can lessen the amount of fat stored. For endomorphs, the usual macronutrient ratio suggestion is 25–30% carbs, 35–40% protein, and 35–40% fat.

Red Blood Cells:
Leafy greens, non-starchy vegetables, and low-sugar fruits are good sources of high-fiber, low-glycemic-index carbs for an endomorph's diet. These carbohydrates can help you feel fuller for longer periods and have less of an effect on blood sugar.

Sermons:

Endomorphs need to consume a lot of protein to support the growth and maintenance of their muscles. Lean meats, seafood, eggs, dairy products, and plant-based foods like tofu, lentils, and beans are all excellent protein sources.

Sizes:
An integral component of the endomorph diet, healthy fats support satiety and energy levels. Avocados, almonds, seeds, olive oil, and fatty fish high in omega-3 fatty acids are good sources of healthful fats.

Time of Meal:
For endomorphs, eating smaller, more frequent meals throughout the day may help to maintain an active metabolism and curb overindulgence. Every meal should contain fiber and protein to help keep blood sugar levels under control and satiety levels intact.

Surfactant:
All body types should maintain proper hydration, but endomorphs should do so even more because water can speed up metabolism and facilitate digestion.

Example Endomorph Meal Plan:

Lunchtime:
- Eggs scrambled with mushrooms and spinach
- An avocado side dish
- Tea Verde

Snack in the Middle of the Morning: - A small portion of berries and a handful of almonds

Peak:
- A salad of grilled chicken or tofu topped with cucumbers, cherry tomatoes, and mixed greens dressed with olive oil
- A complete fruit chunk

Afternoon Snack: - Chia or flaxseeds added to Greek yogurt

Supper:
- Mixed green salad with roasted vegetables, such as broccoli and cauliflower; - Baked fish or lentil stew; - A side dish of roasted veggies

Evening Snack (if needed): - A tiny portion of cottage cheese flavored with cinnamon or a protein shake

Whole, unprocessed foods that supply energy and nutrients without being overly caloric should be the main focus for endomorphs. Endomorphs can achieve their health and fitness objectives and better control their weight by following a diet designed to meet their unique metabolic requirements.

CHARACTERISTICS OF ENDOMORPHS

One of the three main body types is the endomorph, distinguished by a bigger bone structure, a higher amount of body fat, and a tendency to store weight. While every body type has distinctive characteristics and inclinations, endomorphs are frequently identified by their rounder build and difficulties controlling their weight because of their slower metabolism.

Material Properties:
Generally speaking, endomorphs have a soft, curvaceous body type and are more likely than other body types to accumulate fat and muscle. They may have a larger stomach and frequently have shorter limbs. The bodies of endomorphs are better at storing energy, which in the past would have been useful in times of scarcity but can be problematic in the world of abundance we live in now.

Protection:
Compared to ectomorphs or mesomorphs, endomorphs typically burn calories more slowly due to their slower metabolic rates. Because of their slower metabolism, endomorphs find it more difficult to lose fat and must be more careful about their food and exercise regimen to keep their weight in check.

Distribution of Fat and Muscle:
Endomorphs have a larger body fat percentage, which can make it difficult for them to develop well-defined muscles. They frequently accumulate fat in their thighs, hips, and

lower abdomen. Particularly in females, this distribution can occasionally result in a pear-shaped physique.

Action Reaction:
Endomorphs respond well to regular exercise, especially resistance and high-intensity interval training (HIIT), even though they might not lose weight as quickly or readily as other body types. Their naturally sluggish metabolism can be accelerated, and muscle mass can be promoted with these kinds of activities, both of which can help with fat loss.

Needs for Diet:
A diet richer in proteins and fats and lower in carbohydrates frequently benefits endomorphs since it can help control insulin sensitivity and prevent fat buildup. Achieving a stable blood sugar level can be accomplished by consuming smaller meals throughout the day and controlling portion sizes. This can prevent the spikes and crashes that often lead to overeating.

Levels of Energy:
Endomorphs may have erratic energy levels; they frequently feel energized after eating carbs, but as these nutrients are processed by their bodies, they may feel fatigued very rapidly. Keeping their intake of macronutrients in balance can help them maintain their energy levels all day.

Aspects Psychological:
Endomorphs may have problems with body image due to cultural beauty standards that frequently favor a slimmer form. Endomorphs should prioritize their health and functional fitness over cultural norms, which might boost their self-confidence and body image.

Endomorphs can better customize their diet and exercise regimens to meet their demands by being aware of these traits. Endomorphs can reach their fitness and health objectives by concentrating on their advantages, including their capacity for muscular growth, and resolving their disadvantages with a sensible diet and training regimen.

LOW-CARB AND HIGH-PROTEIN STRATEGIES

Whether you consider yourself an endomorph or just discover that your body responds best to a lower-carb, higher-protein diet, you should implement tactics that support these nutritional objectives. You can more effectively manage your weight and body composition by focusing on healthy fats and proteins and consuming fewer carbohydrates.

You'll build each meal, starting with the meals themselves, around a strong protein foundation. Consider lean beef, tofu, tempeh, or grilled chicken breast. You can also try fish like tuna or salmon. In addition to being good for your muscles, these protein sources also boost satiety, which keeps you feeling fuller for longer. Aim for a serving of protein at each meal that is around the size of your hand.

When incorporating carbohydrates, opt for low glycemic index and high fiber content. These will assist in keeping your blood sugar levels stable and prevent the spikes and crashes that can trigger overindulgence in food and hunger. Vegetables like broccoli, cauliflower, and leafy greens should comprise most of your carb sources. You should also include lesser amounts of complex carbohydrates like sweet potatoes or legumes.

You should include good fats in your diet as well. Avocados, nuts & seeds, olive oil, and fatty seafood are good sources. They serve as a slow-burning energy source in addition to being necessary for the synthesis of hormones and the absorption of nutrients.

Regarding dairy, choose low-carb, high-protein options like cottage cheese or Greek yogurt. Several plant-based substitutes are just as high in protein and healthy fats if you must avoid dairy.

To maintain an active metabolism, you must plan out your snacks wisely. Opt for high-protein options like a hard-boiled egg, a cheese stick, or a small handful of nuts instead of chips or crackers. By making these choices, you can avoid insulin spikes caused by high-carb snacks.

Timing your meals is also very important for maintaining the balance of your macronutrients. Eating at regular intervals over the day can assist in controlling your energy and hunger. If you exercise often, eating a mix of carbohydrates and protein before and after your exercises will help you recover from your workouts without going overboard with the carbohydrates.

Finally, always remember to stay hydrated. In addition to boosting your metabolism, drinking water makes it easier for you to distinguish between thirst and hunger. Sometimes, you just need a glass of water instead of an additional snack.

Following these high-protein, low-carb tactics will put you in a position to successfully manage your weight and reach your fitness objectives. Recall that the key is to discover the ideal equilibrium for your particular body type and yourself.

SAMPLE MEAL PLANS AND FOODS

When starting a low-carb, high-protein diet to improve your health, you should concentrate on eating meals that satiate, invigorate, and nourish your body. This is an example of a customized meal plan for you:

Lunchtime:
Start the day off right with a full breakfast. Add a mixture of peppers, mushrooms, and spinach to two scrambled eggs. Enjoy this with some avocado on the side to boost good fats. A protein shake made with almond milk, your preferred protein powder, and a few frozen berries will work wonders if you're on the run.

Lunch in the Middle:
Have a high-protein snack on hand for when the early hunger pangs hit. A tiny container of Greek yogurt topped with almonds offers the ideal balance of crunch and protein.

Peak:
Make a nutrient-dense lunch salad with mixed greens, cucumber, cherry tomatoes, and a hefty portion of grilled chicken or chickpeas for protein. To make a dressing, drizzle some olive oil and vinegar over the salad and top with a little feta cheese for taste.

Dinner Snack:
To keep yourself full and focused until dinner, grab a handful of walnuts or pecans and a piece of low-sugar fruit, such as an apple

or a pear, instead of the vending machine when the afternoon slump arrives.

Supper:
Dinner is a time to relax and treat yourself to a delicious meal. Serve a small piece of quinoa and roasted Brussels sprouts with a grilled salmon fillet or a lentil patty. You won't feel heavy like you would from high-carb meals since the quinoa and salmon's fiber and good fats will keep you full.

Afternoon snack:
Hard-boiled eggs or slices of turkey breast are great options if you crave something small before bed without going overboard with carbohydrates.

Foods You Should Eat:
Make sure to add vegetables that you can eat in large quantities, such as kale, broccoli, and cauliflower, to your shopping list. In addition, it's important to consume high-quality protein sources like fish, fowl, tofu, and lentils. For snacks, reach for nuts and seeds and consider avocados, cheese, and olive oil as your sources of healthy fats.

Although the foods on this list are great for a low-carb, high-protein diet, you should still modify your intake in terms of overall consumption and portion sizes based on your unique energy requirements and health objectives. Always pay attention to your body's signals of hunger and fullness, and modify your meals accordingly. You're well on your way to a well-nourished, balanced day with these meal plans, emphasizing consistency above all else.

PART III: EXERCISE AND LIFESTYLE ADJUSTMENTS FOR EACH BODY TYPE

CHAPTER 7: EXERCISE FOR ECTOMORPHS

Because of your small stature and quick metabolism, ectomorphs must work differently. Your primary goal is to increase muscle mass and strength via a well-organized exercise program that prioritizes resistance training and emphasizes the importance of rest and recovery.

Intense Conditioning:

Heavy, compound workouts like squats, deadlifts, bench presses, and rows should be your top priorities. Multiple muscle groups are worked throughout these exercises, which results in more noticeable strength improvements and an effective workout. Try to get in three to four days a week of strength training, concentrating on challenging yourself with heavier weights for six to ten repetitions. Each exercise must be performed with proper form and maximum effort rather than focusing on quantity.

Intensity and Timing:

Resist the urge to work out every day. Make sure you take at least 48 hours off in between workouts that focus on the same muscle groups because your muscles require this time to grow and heal. This could entail exercising every muscle group once or twice a week but hard enough to promote growth.

Exercise for the Heart:

Although aerobic activity benefits general health, as an

ectomorph, you should avoid doing too much of it since it can lose vital calories needed for muscle growth. To maintain heart health without sacrificing muscle growth, substitute brief, high-intensity interval training (HIIT) sessions or moderate-paced exercise a few times per week.

Flexibility and Mobility Work: Include flexibility and mobility exercises in your program to enhance your strength training. You can decrease your chance of injury, increase muscle recovery, and increase your range of motion with yoga or dynamic stretching. Set aside a minimum of one day per week to concentrate only on this facet of training.

Diet and Recuperation:
The efficacy of your workouts depends on how well you recover. Eat more calories to support muscle growth and exercise. To grow and repair muscle tissue, ensure your diet is well-balanced with fats, proteins, and carbohydrates. Nutrition after exercise is especially crucial, so try to have a high-protein, high-carb meal within 30 minutes of your activity ending.

Regarding Lifestyle:
Getting enough sleep is a must. For the best possible muscle healing and growth hormone release, try to get between seven and nine hours of sleep every night. Additionally, since stress can impede your efforts to gain muscle, learn to control it with conscious techniques like meditation or deep breathing exercises.

Weekly Exercise Schedule Example for Ectomorphs: - Monday: Heavy Upper Body Compound Lifting -Wednesday: Rest or active recovery (yoga or light stretching) - Wednesday: HIIT cardio (20 minutes) - Thursday: Heavy Lower Body Compound Lifting - Friday: 30 minutes of moderately paced cardio - On Saturday, engage in full-body heavy compound lifting.Sunday: Recovery and rest

You're on the right track to developing a more muscular, stronger body that complements your ectomorphic body type if you adhere to these rules. Always pay attention to your body and modify your training and recovery regimen.

BEST TYPES OF EXERCISE FOR ECTOMORPHS

Because of your quick metabolism and lean physique, ectomorphs have a somewhat different wiring when exercising. You must concentrate on particular routines that promote hypertrophy (muscle growth) and strength if you want to see increases in muscle and strength. To prevent burning too many calories or running the risk of overtraining, your routine should be rigorous but not unduly demanding, allowing for sufficient recuperation.

Training in Resistance:
Weightlifting, particularly heavy complex motions that target many muscular groups simultaneously, will be your main focus. Consider performing bench presses, overhead presses, deadlifts, and squats. Your greatest hope for developing size and basic strength is to perform these workouts. Try to lift weights that will test you for three to four sets of six to ten repetitions. The secret is to execute every exercise with correct form and deliberate movements to increase muscle activation and reduce the chance of injury.

Incremental Overload:
You must continuously challenge your muscles by progressively increasing the weight or the amount of repetitions over time if you want to develop bigger and stronger. The idea of progressive loading is essential for ongoing development and muscle growth.

Maintain a training journal to monitor your development, and make sure you're pushing your muscles harder every week, even if it's just a little bit.

Easy Cardio:
Although cardiovascular fitness is vital for general health, as an ectomorph, you should avoid long cardio sessions as they can burn the energy necessary for muscle building. Choose brief, high-intensity interval training (HIIT) sessions instead of lengthier aerobic workouts, as they can enhance cardiovascular health without burning as many calories. It should be enough to do a couple of 20-minute HIIT sessions per week.

Attention to Recovery:
Exercise is important, but so is the recovery period. Ensure you're getting enough sleep and are paying attention to your workouts. Give your muscles time to heal and build since they grow during rest, not exercise. For better flexibility and circulation, aim for 7-9 hours of sleep each night, and think about adding exercises like foam rolling or yoga on your rest days.

Dietary Supplements to Your Workout Program:
Recall that physical activity is only half the fight. For ectomorphs, nutrition is equally crucial. Your muscles will be fueled, and recuperation will be aided by eating adequate calories and concentrating on protein intake before and after workouts. After workouts, think about having a protein shake to help your muscles absorb amino acids faster.

Model Workout Schedule: - Tuesday: HIIT cardio (20 minutes) - Monday: Heavy compound lifting (upper body) - Wednesday: Take a nap or engage in mild exercise, like walking.Friday: HIIT cardio (20 minutes) - Thursday: Heavy compound lifting (lower body) - On Saturday, there will be a full body lifting workout with an emphasis on compound movements.Sunday: Recovery and rest

You may grow the muscle and strength that might not come

as readily to you by working with, rather than against, your ectomorphic qualities by following this exercise plan. Recall that on this path, patience and constancy are your friends.

BUILDING STRENGTH AND MUSCLE MASS

Gaining muscle bulk and strength is a journey that calls for commitment, endurance, and astute training techniques. Prioritize workouts and regimens that will test your muscles and aid in their growth and recuperation as you start along this path.

Pay Attention to Compound Lifts:
Incorporate compound lifts as the first exercise in your regimen. These workouts, which include squats, deadlifts, bench presses, and rows, target several muscular groups simultaneously. Because they let you work multiple muscle groups at once and lift larger weights, they are quite useful for increasing strength. As you gain strength, increase the weight and aim for 4-6 repetitions per set.

Adopt Gradual Overload:
In your pursuit of muscular mass, the concept of progressive overload is essential. This entails building up the weight, frequency, or rep count in your strength training regimen gradually. Give your muscles the stimulus they require to grow by giving them regular challenges. Record your exercise and set a weekly goal to get better.

Make Your Form Perfect:
Make sure you have perfect form before you begin lifting greater weights. To avoid injury and effectively target muscles, proper technique is crucial. Consider hiring a personal trainer to perfect your form. You can also videotape your workouts to review and adjust as needed.

Make Recovery a Priority:
After an exercise, muscles require time to grow and mend. Make sure you're resting for a minimum of 48 hours before working out the same muscle group once more. Include rest days in your schedule, and ensure you get enough sleep—deep sleep is when growth hormone levels are at their highest, which helps with muscle recovery.

Diet is Crucial:
Proper nutrition for your body is equally as crucial as your training schedule. Aim for roughly 1.6 to 2.2 grams of protein per kilogram of body weight while increasing your protein intake to aid muscle rebuilding. Carbs are important because they help you refill your glycogen levels and give you the energy you need to do tough activities. Remember lipids, too, as they are essential for producing hormones, which are necessary for building muscle.

Avoid Dehydration:
When growing muscle, hydration should be more frequently addressed. Water can assist in avoiding weariness and cramping in your muscles and is necessary for transporting nutrients to your muscles. Drink three liters daily if you perspire a lot when working out.

Supplement Carefully: Take into account supplements that promote muscle growth. Popular options that can help you gain muscle are whey protein, creatine, and branched-chain amino acids (BCAAs), especially when combined with a healthy diet.

Example of a Strength-Building Program: Monday: Compound lifts for the upper body (bench press, overhead press) - Tuesday: Compound lifts of the lower body (squats, deadlifts) - Wednesday: Stretching and gentle cardio exercises or rest - Thursday: Strength and hypertrophy of the upper body (pull-ups, rows) - Friday: Strength and hypertrophy of the lower body (leg press, lunges) - Saturday: Core exercises and accessory movements - Sunday:

Complete relaxation

Recall that developing muscle bulk and strength takes time. Your desired outcomes can be achieved through a holistic approach to exercise, recovery, nutrition, and consistent practice over an extended period. As you advance and change, pay attention to your body and be ready to modify your plan.

EXERCISE PLANS AND ROUTINES

Developing an effective fitness regimen involves selecting a routine that will push your body while remaining pleasurable and long-lasting. A well-rounded exercise regimen should include cardiovascular and weight training, flexibility exercises, and enough rest.

Intense Conditioning:
Depending on your objectives and recovery time, you will concentrate on strength training two to four times each week. For a strong foundation, start your workout routine with compound exercises like squats, deadlifts, bench presses, and pull-ups. These exercises work for multiple muscular groups and are highly effective. As you progress, you can move on to isolation exercises that target specific muscles, such as tricep extensions and curls. Always prioritize proper form during your workouts to maximize gains and minimize the risk of injury.

Exercises for the Heart:
Cardio is crucial for both general fitness and heart health. Every week, incorporate one or two cardio exercises. For a more effective, fat-burning workout, try high-intensity interval training (HIIT) instead of steady-state activities like cycling or jogging. If your main objective is to grow muscle, keep your cardio short yet vigorous to prevent burning too many calories.

Mobility and Flexibility: Set aside time to work on mobility and flexibility. This could be accomplished with dynamic stretching, Pilates, or yoga. These exercises increase the range of motion, lower the chance of injury, and speed up muscle recovery. Incorporate at least one weekly session, or think about performing quick stretches right after working out.

Recuperation and Rest:
Days of rest are essential. To enable your muscles to strengthen and heal, schedule one or two full rest days every week at the very least. Additionally, ensure you get a good night's sleep every night because that's when your body heals the most.

Diet and Drinking Water:
Combine a healthy diet with your exercise regimen. To optimize your workouts, consume a well-balanced diet rich in protein, complex carbohydrates, and healthy fats. Stay hydrated by drinking plenty of water throughout the day to enhance your performance.

Regularity and Monitoring of Progress:
The key is consistency. Adhere to your schedule and develop the practice of monitoring your advancement. Keep a workout journal where you may record weight increases, endurance gains, and any modifications to your body composition. This will support your motivation and let you modify your plan as necessary.

Weekly Exercise Schedule Example: - Monday: 15 minutes of HIIT plus upper body strength training - Tuesday: Strength training for the lower body - Wednesday: Rest or gentle yoga to increase range of motion.Thursday: Strength exercise for the entire body - Friday: Core exercises plus cardio (swimming, running, or cycling) - Saturday: Active recuperation (brisk stroll, stretches, or leisure activities) - Sunday: Relax

Always remember that the ideal strategy works with your lifestyle and can be modified in response to your body's needs. Remind yourself that fitness is a lifelong adventure rather than a race, and exercise patience with yourself.

CHAPTER 8: EXERCISE FOR MESOMORPHS

Being a mesomorph means having a robust, muscular body responsive to activity, making you naturally athletic. You have the distinct advantage of being able to reduce fat and increase muscle quite quickly. But to make the most of your genetic potential, you should exercise in a way that enhances your innate personality.

Intense Conditioning:
A healthy combination of cardiovascular and strength training should be part of your fitness routine. To further define your muscles and improve your physique, strength training is essential. Try to lift weights three to four days a week, emphasizing high weights for developing muscle and lighter weights for toning and endurance. Squats, deadlifts, and bench presses are compound exercises that are very beneficial because they engage several muscle groups and provide a powerful stimulus for muscular building.

Exercise for the Heart:
While you don't require as much cardio as an endomorph, it's still necessary for endurance and heart health. Add two to three days of varying-intense cardio to your weekly regimen. Because it highlights your muscle definition and burns a lot of calories quickly, High-Intensity Interval Training (HIIT) can be quite helpful.

Flexibility and Mobility exercises:

Don't overlook flexibility and mobility exercises as part of a well-rounded fitness regimen. By keeping your muscles flexible and elastic, these workouts will lower your chance of injury and enhance your general athletic performance. You should fit in dedicated stretching sessions, Pilates, and yoga as part of your weekly routine.

Recuperation and Rest:
For muscles to grow and recuperate, rest is essential. Ensure you receive one full day of rest per week, at the very least. This is the period when your muscles become bigger and stronger as a result of the micro tears they sustain from lifting weights. Lack of sleep can result in overtraining and progress plateaus.

Diet and Drinking Water:
Your exercise program should be supported by your diet. Your body needs a balanced amount of proteins, lipids, and carbohydrates if you identify as a mesomorph. After a workout, protein is especially crucial for helping muscles recover. Drink plenty of water daily to aid muscle regeneration and metabolic processes.

Weekly Workout Schedule Example for Mesomorphs:
- Monday: Strength training for the upper body and core movements - Tuesday: HIIT workout or cardio at a steady pace - Wednesday: Strength training for the lower body - Thursday: Stretching and gentle cardio for active recovery - Whole body circuit training on FridaySaturday: Cardiovascular endurance (cycling, swimming, walking) - Sunday: Recovery and rest

You can perform well in strength and endurance exercises if you're a mesomorph. You can improve your innate athletic ability and reach your fitness objectives by adhering to an organized training program that consists of a range of routines. To maintain improvement, always pay attention to your body and modify your regimen as necessary.

EFFECTIVE WORKOUTS FOR MESOMORPHS

Your naturally athletic frame as a mesomorph enables you to perform well in various exercises. Making the most of your innate abilities and attending to any areas that require more improvement are your objectives. Here's how to design efficient exercise programs that complement your mesomorphic characteristics.

Intense Conditioning:

With a strength training regimen that includes both big lifts and moderate endurance workouts, you may capitalize on your innate tendency toward muscular gain. Compound exercises, such as squats, bench presses, and deadlifts, involve multiple muscle groups and are great for developing functional strength. Aim to perform them two to three times per week, focusing on challenging yourself with moderate to heavy weights for eight to twelve repetitions. By doing so, you can effectively build your muscles and improve your overall strength.

Use isolation workouts to define and sculpt particular muscular groups, such as tricep dips and curls. To ensure well-rounded muscular growth, these should enhance rather than replace your complex actions.

Training for the Heart:

You'll work out your cardiovascular system with aerobic exercises to maintain cardiovascular health and avoid gaining extra weight. Balance is crucial, too, since you want to stay moderate and maintain the muscular mass you've worked so hard to develop. To optimize effectiveness and fat burning, do two to three days of cardio, alternating between high-intensity interval training (HIIT) and steady-state activities like cycling or running.

Agility Training and Plyometrics:
Make the most of your innate athleticism by including agility and plyometric training. Exercises that increase explosive power and speed, such as box jumps, jump squats, and ladder drills, can enhance your strength development.

Main Task:
Performance and overall fitness depend heavily on a robust core. Incorporate exercises that work your entire core—not just your abs. Leg raises, Russian twists, and planks are workouts that will assist in strengthening and stabilizing the core, which will aid with all other exercises and daily tasks.

Adaptability and Movement:
Pay attention to the significance of mobility and flexibility. Stretching should be done dynamically during warm-ups and statically during cool-downs to help you retain a complete range of motion and lower your chance of injury. To further improve your flexibility, consider adding Pilates or yoga to your weekly practice.

Healing:
Give your recuperation the same priority as your workouts. Even though mesomorphs tend to heal more quickly than other body types, getting enough sleep is still crucial. Every week, give yourself at least one full day off and think about employing massage or foam rolling to help your muscles heal.

Weekly Workout Plan Example:
- Monday: Core stability exercises and heavy compound lifting
- Tuesday: Sprint intervals or HIIT -Wednesday: Intense recuperation (brisk walk or swim) - Thursday: Agility and

plyometric workouts - Friday: Core strengthening and upper body isolation exercises - Saturday: Extended cardio workout at a steady state - Sunday: Recovery and rest

By following this exercise plan, you may maximize your mesomorphic advantages and ensure that your muscles remain defined and functioning, your cardiovascular fitness remains high, and you gain strength. Always pay attention to your body's needs and modify as needed, particularly if you feel you're overtraining or need more sleep.

FOCUS ON TONING AND FLEXIBILITY

Include high repetitions of lighter-weight workouts to tone your body and improve your flexibility. This method emphasizes the definition and endurance of the muscles. Include exercises that target various muscle groups. For example, pair lunges with bicep curls or squats with shoulder presses. Aim for 12–15 repetitions with a modest weight.

Including workouts using your own weight is also crucial for toning. Perform exercises such as push-ups, planks, leg lifts, and mountain climbers to simultaneously work several muscle groups. Without gaining size, these exercises are good for shaping muscles.

Including yoga in your exercise routine will help you become much more flexible. Yoga's different poses and stretches, particularly those from Vinyasa or Hatha styles, lengthen and stretch your muscles, which helps you recuperate and seem thinner.

You should incorporate dynamic stretches into your warm-up regimen. They increase the range of motion and prime your joints and muscles for the upcoming activity. Incorporate arm circles, leg swings, and twisting lunges, among other exercises.

Use stability equipment like balance balls and incorporate exercises like planks and Russian twists to develop core strength and balance, which are crucial for toning. These help with everyday motions by strengthening your core and overall balance.

Additionally, cardiovascular activity contributes to toning. It aids in shedding any excess fat and can highlight the desired muscular definition. Pick enjoyable aerobic activities to enhance your toning efforts, such as swimming, cycling, or brisk walking.

It is essential to set aside time for stretching after vigorous exercise. This can help avoid muscle tension and will facilitate recuperation. All of the main muscle groups should be the focus of your stretches, and you should pay special attention to any places that seem very tight or painful.

Aim for a weekly mix of light cardio, core workouts, flexibility work, and high-repetition strength training. This may be as simple as doing a circuit training session one day, then stretching or yoga the next, cardio with core work, and Pilates or toning classes after that. Include days dedicated to gentle activities like walking or restorative yoga because active recuperation is just as vital.

It is important to include toning exercises and flexibility training in your weekly routine. This will help you achieve a more defined physique, improve your overall fitness, reduce the risk of injuries, and increase your range of motion for various physical activities. Consistency is key to seeing results, so stick to your routine. It is also important to listen to your body and find a healthy balance between work and relaxation.

EXERCISE PLANS AND ROUTINES

Starting a fitness journey means creating a detailed strategy that works for your objectives and way of life. Start off by doing strength training two to four times a week, concentrating on compound exercises that target several muscle groups. Your regimen will consist primarily of exercises like bench presses and squats, which will help you develop a strong foundation. To improve muscle endurance and definition, combine greater repetitions with lesser weights when toning. Make sure you're pushing your muscles to fatigue.

Include cardiovascular exercises to promote fat loss and maintain the health of your heart. You can opt for more strenuous, effective workouts like high-intensity interval training (HIIT) or steady-state workouts like cycling or walking. Two to three aerobic activities per week should be plenty to achieve balance, as long as you don't burn out or lose muscle mass while burning calories.

You shouldn't undervalue flexibility and mobility because they complete your fitness and help you avoid injuries. Schedule time for dynamic stretching or yoga; these should be a crucial component of your warm-up and cool-down exercises. Your range of motion will increase, which will help you perform better in other activities.

Keep in mind how important sleep is. Your muscles can repair and strengthen if you take at least one day off each week. To guarantee that you're well-rested and prepared for each workout, sleep is another essential component of your recovery process. Aim for seven to nine hours each night.

Your exercise regimen should be complemented by your diet. Ensure your body gets the proper amounts of lipids, proteins, and carbohydrates; in particular, pay attention to how much protein you eat to support muscle growth and repair. It's important to drink water regularly throughout the day to maintain hydration levels and enhance performance. Please make sure to check for any spelling, grammar, or punctuation errors.

Exercise consistently, but allow yourself to be adaptable as well. Pay attention to your body; if you're feeling exhausted, take it easy and concentrate on getting better. Maintain a training journal in which you may monitor your development and make any corrections. This will assist you in staying on course and allowing you to observe your progress over time.

Include weightlifting and bodyweight exercises in your weekly regimen, aerobic activities, and time for flexibility and stretching. This could be lifting a lot of weight one day, doing a HIIT workout the next, and setting out a day for yoga or stretching. Make sure to schedule rest days to give your body time to heal.

You're putting yourself in a successful position by creating a well-rounded fitness program with various exercises. Whether you want to enhance your general health, boost endurance, or build strength, this technique will help you reach your fitness objectives. Remember that everyone's road to fitness is unique and dynamic, so adjust your regimen to suit your needs and those of your body.

CHAPTER 9: EXERCISE FOR ENDOMORPHS

Your workout regimen should be designed to maximize fat burning, improve muscle tone, and enhance general metabolic health if you're an endomorph looking to get fit. Because of the tendency of your body type to store fat, you will concentrate on activities that will increase your metabolism and help you get a leaner physique.

Your schedule will include a lot of cardiovascular activities. Exercises that are good for burning calories and reducing fat include rowing, swimming, cycling, and brisk walking. You may benefit most from high-intensity interval training (HIIT) because it increases your metabolism during and for hours following physical activity—a phenomenon called the "afterburn effect." Try to get 3–4 cardio workouts per week, but pay attention to your body to prevent overdoing it.

Take advantage of strength training, though. Cardio helps burn fat, but building muscle requires strength training, which can raise your resting metabolic rate. Concentrate on full-body workouts that use movements like squats, deadlifts, and push-ups to target several muscle groups. To increase your muscular mass and endurance, combine moderate weights with increased repetition counts. Try to fit in two or three strength training sessions every week.

By fusing strength and cardio into a single, effective workout, circuit training may give you the best of both worlds. Create circuits that alternate between brief cardio bursts and resistance training, with little time spent at rest to sustain a fast heart rate.

Exercises for mobility and flexibility should also be a regular routine component. Your flexibility will increase with yoga or pilates, which will help you conduct strength training with the correct form and lower your chance of injury. These practices can also have a relaxing impact, which can aid in stress management, which frequently results in emotional eating.

Ensure your weekly schedule includes at least one complete rest day to guarantee proper recuperation. Your exercise regimen must include recovery for your muscles to heal and strengthen. Light exercise on your rest day, such as rejuvenating yoga or a leisurely stroll, can help your muscles heal and keep you moving without overstressing your body.

Remember that eating right and exercising regularly are equally vital. To feed your body and promote recuperation, combine your workouts with a well-balanced meal high in proteins, healthy fats, and low-glycemic carbohydrates.

Cardiovascular activity, strength training, flexibility training, and adequate rest will help you develop a well-rounded program that promotes weight loss, increased muscle tone, and better metabolic health. Exercise consistently and have patience; the desired effects will manifest themselves in due course.

CARDIOVASCULAR AND FAT-BURNING EXERCISES

A well-planned combination of activities will maximize your body's potential as you work to improve your cardiovascular health and lose fat. Your goal should be to engage in activities that raise and sustain your heart rate in the fat-burning zone, which is normally between 60 and 70 percent of your maximal heart rate.

Begin with steady-state aerobic exercises like swimming, cycling, jogging, or brisk walking. These longer-duration exercises are great for increasing endurance—lasting anywhere from thirty to an hour. They can be a terrific method to get your body moving and are very effective at burning fat when done regularly, especially if you're just starting out with a fitness regimen.

But you'll also include high-intensity interval training (HIIT) to kick-start fat loss. With HIIT, there are brief intervals of high-intensity exercise or relaxation between periods of lower-intensity activity. Your metabolism can be significantly impacted, for instance, by running for thirty seconds, walking for one minute, and continuing this cycle for fifteen to twenty minutes. This kind of training raises your metabolic rate for hours after the workout, in addition to burning many calories during it.

Remember that circuit training can incorporate aspects of both aerobic and strength training, offering a complete exercise that both burns calories and increases muscle. Jumping jacks, burpees, push-ups, and squats could all be performed in a circuit, one after the other, with little to no break between sets. This challenges every part of your body and maintains an elevated heart rate.

Rowing is an additional efficient aerobic and fat-burning workout. Using up most of the body's muscles, cardio burns calories and is low-impact, being kinder to joints.

Incorporate exciting techniques to increase heart rate and burn calories, such as kickboxing or dance exercise courses, into your regimen. These workouts have the power to improve your mood and are frequently so entertaining that you won't even realize you're exercising.

Remember that your body adjusts to exercise with time, so to keep pushing yourself and avoid hitting a plateau in your fat reduction journey, switch up your activities. Additionally, adjust the length and intensity of your workouts to your goals and fitness level and allow enough time for rest and recovery.

It's important to combine these workouts with a healthy diet and adequate water to meet your energy requirements and promote your body's recovery. Additionally, pay close attention to your body's needs, and always adjust the intensity and duration of your workouts according to your ability and how you feel. With commitment and perseverance, you can reduce your body fat and improve your cardiovascular health.

STRENGTH TRAINING AND BODY COMPOSITION

Strength training has a major impact on your total body composition in addition to helping you gain muscle. Gaining more muscular mass, strength, and endurance through resistance training is the aim of strength training. It has a significant impact on body composition since it raises lean muscle mass, which raises metabolic rate and lowers body fat percentage.

Strength training is a great way to change your body composition since it pushes your muscles beyond their limits. This is using weights that are heavy enough that you can only complete a predetermined amount of repetitions before experiencing muscular fatigue; typically, this is between 8 and 12 repetitions for hypertrophy (muscle growth) or between 4 and 6 repetitions for maximum strength improvements.

Exercises that are considered compound include overhead presses, bench presses, squats, and deadlifts. These exercises are highly effective for developing strength and muscle because they engage several muscle groups simultaneously. Additionally, they mimic actions and motions seen in the real world, which enhances functional strength.

By switching up your strength training sessions between days with greater lifts and days with lighter, higher repetitions, you may provide variation to your program. This method, called periodization, can lower your risk of overuse injuries and help you avoid reaching progress plateaus. You challenge your muscles to get stronger on heavier days and to get more muscle endurance on lighter days.

Recall that the amount of weight lifted matters less than the quality of the action. To maximize your results and prevent injuries, maintain good form. To get your technique right, working with a trainer at first is beneficial.

Exercises alone are not as crucial as rest and recuperation. Because muscles require time to grow and heal, you'll ensure your routine includes rest days. Your body builds muscle when you're at rest, gradually changing the makeup of your body.

When it comes to body composition and strength training, nutrition is essential. You'll concentrate on getting adequate protein for muscle growth and repair, carbs for energy during exercise, and healthy fats for general health support. Water supports all bodily processes, including the development and repair of muscles; therefore, staying hydrated is also essential.

Track your development about changes in body composition as well as strength gains. This might inspire you and let you know if your present routine is working or needs to be adjusted.

You can improve your body composition by increasing muscle mass and reducing body fat through proper strength training, healthy eating, and rest. This improves your overall health and metabolism and your physical attractiveness. Remind yourself to be patient with yourself because it takes time and persistent effort to change your body composition.

EXERCISE PLANS AND ROUTINES

If you are an endomorph, your fitness regimen should focus on increasing your metabolism, decreasing body fat, and developing lean muscle. You'll concentrate on exercises that increase your body's capacity to burn fat because your body type inherently stores fat and conserves energy.

Cardiovascular Exercises:

Begin with a cardiovascular workout. You'll gain from high-intensity interval training (HIIT) and steady-state cardio exercises like brisk walking, swimming, or cycling. Regularly doing high-intensity interval training (HIIT) can assist you in burning a significant amount of calories swiftly and maintaining a fast metabolism even after you finish exercising. According to health guidelines, it is suggested to aim for 150 minutes of moderate-intensity or 75 minutes of high-intensity cardio exercises every week for optimal results.

Intense Exercise:

At least twice or three times a week, including weight training in your regimen. Exercises that train many muscle parts simultaneously, such as squats, deadlifts, and bench presses, should be your main focus. These exercises can help you gain muscular mass, enhancing your resting metabolic rate. Remember that, even when at rest, you will burn more calories if you have greater muscle.

Circuit Instruction:

Circuit exercise is especially beneficial. Strength training combines quick cardio bursts to increase heart rate and burn more calories. Create circuits using a range of exercises that focus on various muscle groups and switch between workouts for the core, lower body, and upper body.

Mobility and Flexibility:
Remember to incorporate workouts for mobility and flexibility into your regimen. Your range of motion is improved, your risk of injury is decreased, and you can perform better in other exercises by engaging in yoga or pilates. Additionally, it keeps your joints and muscles healthy and balances the high-intensity work you do.

Recovery and Rest: Schedule enough time for recuperation and rest. Exercise is a great way for endomorphs to work hard, but rest is when your body heals and strengthens. Plan one or two days off each week, and make sure you're getting enough sleep every night.

Example Weekly Workout Schedule for Endomorphs:
- Tuesday: Full-body strength training - Monday: HIIT workout or brisk walking -Wednesday: Swimming and cycling at a moderate effort - Thursday: Rest or mild yoga - Friday: Circuit training combining cardio and weight training - Saturday: HIIT training or athletic engagement - Sunday: relaxation or active recuperation (brisk stroll, stretches)

Never forget to provide your body with the nutrition for exercise —a balanced meal high in fiber, protein, and healthy fats. It's also crucial to stay hydrated. By adhering to this approach, you will tackle the endomorph's obstacles and work towards increasing your body's inherent capabilities. Recall that tiny daily efforts over time result in significant results, and constancy is essential.

PART IV: INTEGRATING MIND-BODY WELLNESS

CHAPTER 10: MINDFULNESS AND WEIGHT LOSS

Practicing mindfulness can greatly enhance your ability to balance your physical and mental well-being, making it an invaluable tool in your weight reduction journey. Along this journey, it's not only about what you put in your mouth or how much exercise you get in; it's also about developing a greater understanding of your body's demands, your emotional triggers, and the habits that mold your everyday existence.

By incorporating mindfulness into your weight reduction routine, you'll be more attentive to the decisions you make about your diet and level of physical activity. To avoid overindulging and enjoy the sensation of being nourished, it's essential to eat mindfully and pay close attention to the flavors and textures of your food. By being more aware of your eating, you can control your portion sizes and improve your comprehension of fullness and hunger signals.

Being alert One of the mainstays of your weight loss attempts can be meditation. You can improve your emotional resilience and stress management—two things that are frequently connected to weight gain—by engaging in regular meditation practice. Reducing stress can help prevent emotional eating, and meditation fosters a calm state of mind that facilitates thoughtful meal selection.

Exercises that connect your body and mind while burning calories are another way to incorporate mindfulness into your physical activity. Exercises that focus on breath and movement and help you stay anchored in the present moment, such as yoga and tai chi, are ideal for this. This can make working out more enjoyable, transforming it from duty into something more fulfilling that you eagerly anticipate.

Sleep is another component of mindfulness in weight loss. You'll emphasize proper sleep hygiene routines when you take a conscious approach. You can enhance the balance of your hormones, especially those that control hunger, such as ghrelin and leptin, by obtaining enough good sleep.

Beyond the dinner table, mindful eating includes grocery shopping and meal preparation. Rather than eating on the spur of the moment or for convenience, you'll shop mindfully, selecting foods that support your health and preparing meals that fill you up.

You'll consider the emotional components of eating as well. You can identify trends that might impede weight loss by analyzing the emotions influencing your eating choices. By accepting these behaviors without passing judgment, you can start forming new, more wholesome routines.

Including mindfulness in your weight reduction journey entails a more comprehensive well-being approach. It's about developing a way of life that respects your body's requirements and lets you lose weight compassionately and mindfully. Throughout this chapter, you will discover methods for developing your mindfulness practice and applying these ideas to various facets of your life, ultimately resulting in a well-rounded strategy for both weight reduction and general well-being wellbeing.

THE ROLE OF MINDFULNESS AND MEDITATION

Beyond customary practices, mindfulness and meditation have a huge part in modern life. By inviting you to experience the present moment without passing judgment, mindfulness challenges you to live in a society where multitasking and digital distractions are the norm. This structured practice of meditation can significantly improve both physical and mental well-being.

By focusing on your present experiences, mindfulness training helps you develop an awareness that can change how you interact with the outside world. It teaches you to step back and analyze your thoughts and feelings without categorizing them as positive or negative. Because you're less prone to respond impulsively or fall victim to negative thought patterns, this helps promote emotional stability.

During meditation, you may choose to concentrate on your breathing, a mantra, or your physical sensations. This concentrated attention helps ease mental tension and calm the psyche. Regular stress is a major cause of many health problems, and you can enhance your general health by using meditation as a stress management technique.

Meditation and mindfulness have been connected to better immunological function, reduced blood pressure, and better sleep in terms of physical health. The body's relaxation response, triggered during meditation, is the source of these advantages. Healing and restoration occur during this response, the opposite of the fight-or-flight reaction.

Additionally important to behavior change are mindfulness and meditation, which are especially important if you want to give up bad habits and develop better ones. It is possible to break the automatic pattern of conduct that results in unhealthful decisions by increasing your awareness of your impulses. Change occurs in this space between impulse and action.

You can improve your eating experiences by practicing mindfulness. Eating mindfully involves savoring each bite, paying attention to hunger and fullness cues, and avoiding overeating to strengthen your relationship with food.

Additionally, meditation might help you develop a closer relationship with yourself. It provides an area for introspection, which is quite beneficial for comprehending the reasons behind your behavior. When planning and establishing objectives for one's profession, personal development, or health, self-awareness is essential.

It has been demonstrated that mindfulness meditation is a useful adjunctive treatment for people who are depressed or anxious. By encouraging a sense of calm and disengagement from upsetting thoughts, it can lessen the symptoms of sadness and anxiety.

It takes less than hours to incorporate mindfulness and meditation into your daily practice. Benefits can be obtained from even little sessions, such as five to ten minutes daily. Your brain clarity, stress levels, emotional well-being, and general outlook on life may change significantly due to these practices over time.

Your experience with mindfulness and meditation will probably lead to a greater sense of calm, mental clarity, and appreciation for every moment as you practice these practices. This change in viewpoint can improve all facets of your life and well-being.

STRESS REDUCTION TECHNIQUES

Having efficient stress management techniques at your disposal can help you deal with the constant demands of modern life and preserve your well-being. To counterbalance the stress-induced fight-or-flight response, begin with deep, diaphragmatic breathing. This initiates your body's relaxation response. To promote calmness, take a deep breath, let your belly rise, hold it for a little while, and gently release it.

Another method is progressive muscle relaxation, in which each muscle group is systematically tense and then released. This improves body awareness and releases tension.

Visualize calm situations or tales to participate in guided imagery. You can find calmness and a distraction from your worries by going on this mental vacation. You can complete these visualization exercises with a plethora of digital tools.

It can also be quite advantageous to incorporate mindfulness meditation into your regular practice. One way to develop a mindfulness practice that will assist you in managing life's stressors in a composed and collected manner is to sit quietly and concentrate on your breathing or a repeating sound.

Regular physical activity should be incorporated into your life as an effective stress reliever. Exercise not only boosts endorphins, which are natural mood enhancers but also helps you shift your focus from daily concerns. To make it a regular part of your routine, select an activity that you enjoy.

Yoga and tai chi combine physical poses, breathing exercises, and meditation to reduce stress and promote relaxation, offering a range of benefits for physical and mental health.

You should always appreciate the significance of social support. One way to reduce stress is to spend time with loved ones, participate in community activities, or get professional help. Furthermore, stress can be avoided by practicing good time management. Prioritize your work, make realistic goals, and practice saying no when appropriate.

Maintaining a journal can help you understand and process your thoughts and feelings, which can be a therapeutic method to deal with stress. This may help you identify the sources of your life's stress and offer some possible remedies.

Calming aromatherapy, like as lavender, can also contribute to the creation of a relaxing environment in which to relax. For their calming effects, incorporate incense, scented candles, or essential oils into your daily routine.

Getting enough sleep is essential for reducing stress. Create a peaceful bedtime routine and comfortable sleeping environment to improve sleep quality.

You will develop a thorough stress management routine by incorporating these approaches into your daily routine. You can find the tactics that work best for you via trial and error, but consistent practice is the key to long-term stress relief and improving your quality of life in general.

MIND-BODY EXERCISES FOR ALL BODY TYPES

For all body types, mind-body activities are a vital part of a holistic approach to health and wellness. These exercises increase mental clarity and reduce stress by relaxing the mind and toning and strengthening the body.

Whether you're an endomorph, mesomorph, or ectomorph, mind-body exercises can be customized to fit your specific requirements and are an added bonus to your current exercise regimen.

Yoga is a flexible exercise suitable for all body types. Yoga offers moderate stretches and positions that aid with stress reduction and flexibility. Yoga can help ectomorphs develop muscle awareness and strength, which may not come naturally. Mesomorphs can utilize yoga to increase their flexibility and strength, which may be lacking in their muscular physique. Yoga may benefit endomorphs in reducing weight, increasing flexibility, and managing stress.

Another mind-body workout that promotes muscular balance, good posture, and core strength is Pilates. Building a solid foundation is especially advantageous, as it is essential for all body types. Pilates can assist mesomorphs in keeping their muscular balance and flexibility, endomorphs in toning their bodies and increasing their metabolic rate, and ectomorphs in developing strength and core stability.

Tai Chi, sometimes called "meditation in motion," is a slow-moving, low-impact workout based on mindfulness and deep breathing. Both endomorphs and ectomorphs benefit from it in terms of stress management and increased attention. Tai Chi is a good way for mesomorphs, who find it tranquil, to balance out their usually hard workouts.

Qigong enhances the body's energy flow through postures and motions combined with rhythmic breathing. Your body's energy can be more harmoniously balanced with this practice, enhancing your health and energy. Increasing your stamina with low-impact exercise can help manage weight and stress.

Including these mind-body exercises in your regimen will help you become more conscious of your body, regardless of shape. They advise paying attention to how your body feels when performing the exercises, which can help you remember to use the right muscles when working out. Enhanced consciousness can also result in improved alignment and posture throughout daily tasks.

In addition to helping you achieve your fitness objectives, these exercises also foster mindfulness, which can assist you in making more deliberate decisions about your diet and way of life. Engaging in mindfulness techniques can assist you in being more aware of your body's signals of hunger and fullness, which can lessen the chance that you would overeat out of emotion. This is especially useful if you are having trouble controlling your weight.

These activities can also have a major positive impact on mental health. They have been shown to lessen depressive and anxious symptoms, enhance the quality of sleep, and uplift mood in general. The overall enhancement of your mental well-being might benefit your physical well-being and fitness objectives.

Including mind-body exercises in your regimen doesn't take long; even a few minutes might be helpful. Maintaining consistency is essential to fully benefit from this approach, and you should observe gains in your mental and emotional well-being and physical health over time.

CHAPTER 11: OVERCOMING WEIGHT LOSS PLATEAUS

You may experience a plateau in your weight reduction journey when the scale stays where it is no matter how hard you try. It's a typical and annoying experience, but you can get past it and keep moving toward your objectives if you take the appropriate strategy.

First, realize that hitting a plateau in your weight loss efforts is common. Your body needs less calories to operate when you lose weight than it did when you were heavier. Weight loss may stall if your exercise regimen and calorie consumption have yet to be modified to consider this.

Considering your present weight, reevaluate your calorie requirements. Your calorie need for weight maintenance has dropped along with your weight loss. To make sure you're not overeating, use an updated BMR calculator.

Next, assess your eating patterns. Are you keeping proper track of the calories you consume? Over time, extra bites, bigger servings, or inaccurate calorie counts may creep in. Return to tracking everything you eat, including the smallest snack or condiment, and make sure you're recording it all.

It's also critical to think about the caliber of your calorie intake.

Your body will be fuelled more efficiently by nutrient-dense foods than by empty calories from processed foods. It is important to maintain a balanced diet that includes whole foods, such as whole grains, fruits, and vegetables, as well as lean proteins.

Change up the way you work out. Over time, your body adjusts to repeated exertion, increasing its efficiency and lowering its caloric expenditure. You can rekindle weight loss by pushing your body harder during exercises or experimenting with other kinds of exercise. If you haven't already, think about adding strength training because it can raise your metabolic rate due to increased muscle mass.

Recall the significance of recuperation and rest. Hormonal imbalances brought on by prolonged stress and sleep deprivation may make it more difficult to lose weight. To help you lose weight, learn stress-reduction strategies and make sure you're getting enough good sleep.

Water is another important yet frequently ignored factor. There are instances when what seems to be hunger is really thirst. Remaining well hydrated will help you prevent mindless munching.

If, despite following all of these suggestions, you find yourself at a standstill, speak with a dietician or other medical expert. They can offer additional tactics that are suited to your circumstances and assist in identifying any underlying problems that might be impeding your weight loss.

Finally, exercise perseverance and patience. It's not always linear to lose weight, and plateaus are simply momentary obstacles. If you stick to your healthy routines, you'll have a better chance of progressing toward your objectives.

IDENTIFYING AND OVERCOMING PLATEAUS

You've reached a plateau when your weight loss efforts completely halt. It's a stage when weight doesn't change, even when you follow a diet or fitness regimen. To surmount this obstacle, one must comprehend its origins and execute tactical adjustments.

Reevaluate your calorie consumption first. Your metabolic rate will often decrease when you lose weight because your body becomes more efficient at using energy. As a result, you might need to consume more calories now to maintain your current weight than when you were trying to lose weight. To be sure you're still in a deficit, recalculate your daily calorie needs using your new weight.

Examine your eating patterns after that. Over time, it's simple to let excess calories creep in. Are you approximating or precisely measuring your portions? Are you ignoring any hidden calories in sauces, dressings, or drinks? You should track your consumption with honesty and precision.

Examine the caliber of your diet. It is preferable to fuel your body with nutrient-dense foods as opposed to high in calories. Most of your diet should consist of lean meats, whole grains, fruits, and vegetables. Foods high in fiber and protein prolong feelings of fullness, making them beneficial for weight loss.

Change up the way you exercise. Your body has grown accustomed to the same training regimen if you've been doing it for weeks or months. It's essential to switch up your workout routine every few weeks to challenge your body. This can include increasing the intensity of your workouts, adding resistance training, or varying your cardio.

Think about getting enough rest and recuperating. Reducing body weight requires both stress management and getting enough sleep. High-stress levels can cause the release of chemicals like cortisol, which is linked to fat storage, and poor sleep can increase appetite and hunger.

Verify that you are consuming adequate water. Maintaining proper hydration is essential for metabolism and appetite regulation. The body might occasionally misinterpret signals of hunger for those of dehydration, causing overeating when water is actually needed.

Should your plateau continue, consulting a healthcare provider may be worthwhile. Your weight reduction stall may have medical causes, such as metabolic disorders or hormone imbalances, which require expert care.

Above all, it takes patience. Plateaus are a normal aspect of weight loss; it's an ups-and-down trip. Remain dedicated, practice self-compassion, and concentrate on the improvements you're making to your health. You should overcome the plateau and get closer to your weight loss objectives with patience and perseverance.

ADJUSTING DIET AND EXERCISE

When you hit a weight reduction plateau, it's usually important to adjust your food and exercise regimen. Your body changes with time, and so do its needs for nutrition and exercise. To break through a plateau, you must carefully evaluate your present routine.

Start by giving your diet another look. As you lose weight, your calorie requirements decrease since a smaller body uses less energy to sustain. It's important to reevaluate your daily calorie consumption based on weight, age, and activity level. Make sure to keep a calorie deficit without becoming unhealthy or unmanageable.

Consider what you eat in addition to how much of it. Your meals should be centered around nutrient-dense foods, such as fruits, vegetables, whole grains, lean meats, and healthy fats. These meals give your body the vitamins and minerals it needs and help you feel fuller for longer periods, which can help you resist mindless munching.

Controlling portion sizes is essential because, when consumed in excess, even healthful meals can add to a calorie surplus. To guarantee precise portion proportions, consider measuring devices or a food scale. Furthermore, be mindful of caloric creep, the steady rise in calorie intake that can happen without your awareness.

It is equally important to refine your training plan and make dietary adjustments. Suppose you've been working out consistently for a long time. In that case, your body might have become accustomed to it, making it less efficient for losing weight. To push your body in novel ways, add new exercises, lengthen or intensify your routines, or switch up the activity you perform.

Gaining muscle mass through strength training is especially beneficial for raising resting metabolic rate. You can change the resistance type, weight, number of repetitions and sets, and pace of exercises even if you are already undertaking strength training.

Think about modifying not just your physical appearance but also when you eat and exercise. To keep your metabolism going, eat smaller, more frequent meals throughout the day. Planning your carbohydrate diet to coincide with your workouts can help you repair your muscles afterward and provide you the energy you need to work out.

Remain hydrated; water aids in weight management and is necessary for metabolic activities. Being well-hydrated can help you avoid overeating because sometimes dehydration is confused with hunger.

See a nutritionist or personal trainer for advice if these changes are ineffective. They can offer a more customized and thorough plan made to meet the unique requirements of your body.

Lastly, exercise patience. It's common for weight reduction to be nonlinear, and plateaus are a normal—if annoying— aspect of the process. You can overcome obstacles and keep moving toward your weight loss objectives with cautious changes and a dedication to your general well-being. Recall that changing to a healthier lifestyle is the goal, not merely a lower weight on the scale.

STAYING MOTIVATED

When your weight loss efforts plateau, it might put your motivation to the test. It's critical to develop strategies to maintain your commitment to your health goals during these times. While motivation varies from person to person and is always changing, there are ways to stay positive and focused.

First, change the way you think. A plateau is your body's way of adjusting to the changes you've made, not a sign of failure. This is a sign of progress to be encouraged to review and adjust your plan. Take the challenge as a chance for personal development.

Review and rephrase your objectives. If losing weight has been your main goal, think about creating performance-based objectives like lifting a certain weight or running a certain distance. These objectives can provide one with a sense of accomplishment independent of magnitude.

Honor the successes that don't have a pound value. Your energy has increased, your sleep has improved, or your mood has improved. Recognizing these non-scale successes can help you stay motivated and remind you of the advantages of leading a healthy lifestyle beyond weight reduction.

Make connections with people who have similar objectives to yours. Encouragement might be found in joining an online group, taking fitness classes, or traveling with a friend. You may stay involved and accountable by sharing your achievements, setbacks, and experiences with others.

To keep things interesting, change up your routine. Rekindling your passion for exercise might be achieved by taking a new sport or fitness class. For healthy eating, new dishes or a culinary class might have the same effect. Sustaining your motivation can be achieved by keeping your trip interesting.

Establish attainable short-term goals that help you get to your long-term objective. These benchmarks ought to be quantifiable and practical. Reaching these minor goals will help you feel like you're making progress all the time and keep you going.

Imagine yourself succeeding. Every day, take some time to visualize achieving your objectives. Using visualization, you may strengthen your subconscious mind's focus on achievement and dedication to your objectives.

Give yourself a reward when you reach your short-term goals. Select incentives that honor your dedication without impeding your advancement: a massage, a movie night, or a new training attire are some ideas.

Learn about diet and health. Knowing the science behind your efforts will help you overcome difficulties with fresh ideas and emphasize how important it is to follow through on your strategy.

Remember your initial motivation. Remember why you started this adventure in the first place. When you start to lose motivation, go over them in writing.

Finally, practice self-compassion. Everyone has disappointments in life. Instead of self-criticism, cultivate self-compassion. Remember that persistence is essential and that development is rarely linear.

It's important to remember that reaching a weight loss plateau calls for a combination of goal reevaluation, non-scale victory celebration, community engagement, and constant reminders of the greater motivations driving your quest for health. Using these techniques, you can overcome obstacles and maintain motivation even when faced with plateaus.

CONCLUSION

Embracing Your Unique Weight Loss Journey

It's important to acknowledge and celebrate the distinct route you take on the road to improved health when you embrace your unique weight loss experience. Your journey, molded by your experiences, body type, and personal objectives, is as unique as your fingerprint. It's a journey that imparts lessons on exercise, diet, and self-improvement in addition to personal growth.

Recognize that it's okay if what works for someone else doesn't work for you. It is important to consider how your body reacts to dietary and exercise changes because it is unique. It makes sense to adapt your strategy to your needs, interests, and way of life; in fact, it's essential for long-term success.

Recognize that losing weight is not always a linear process. Setbacks and plateaus are normal parts of the process; they are not obstacles to success but chances to improve your approach. They inspire you to cultivate traits that benefit you beyond physical well-being, such as patience, resilience, and flexibility.

Honor your accomplishments, regardless of how minor they may appear. Every step you take to advance toward your ultimate objective is a win. Concurrently, take lessons from the difficulties. These important lessons frequently help you become more self-aware and comprehend your body more deeply.

Above all, remember that your weight reduction journey is about creating a healthier, happier life rather than just losing weight. Committing to taking care of oneself can result in significant changes on the inside and out, both mentally and physically. Every step you take will be a step toward becoming a better version of yourself if you embrace the adventure with an open heart and compassion.

CELEBRATING INDIVIDUAL ACHIEVEMENTS

It's important to acknowledge and celebrate the distinct route you take on the road to improved health when you embrace your unique weight loss experience. Your journey, molded by your experiences, body type, and personal objectives, is as unique as your fingerprint. It's a journey that imparts lessons on exercise, diet, and self-improvement in addition to personal growth.

Recognize that it's okay if what works for someone else doesn't work for you. It is important to consider how your body reacts to dietary and exercise changes because it is unique. It makes sense to adapt your strategy to your needs, interests, and way of life; in fact, it's essential for long-term success.

Recognize that losing weight is not always a linear process. Setbacks and plateaus are normal parts of the process; they are not obstacles to success but chances to improve your approach. They inspire you to cultivate traits that benefit you beyond physical well-being, such as patience, resilience, and flexibility.

Honor your accomplishments, regardless of how minor they may appear. Every step you take to advance toward your ultimate objective is a win. Concurrently, take lessons from the difficulties. These important lessons frequently help you become more self-aware and comprehend your body more deeply.

Above all, never forget that your weight reduction journey is about creating a healthier, happier life rather than just losing weight. Committing to taking care of oneself can result in significant changes on the inside and out, both mentally and physically. Every step you take will be a step toward becoming a better version of yourself if you embrace the adventure with an open heart and compassion.

CONTINUING THE PATH TO HEALTH AND WELLNESS

Pursuing health and well-being wellbeing is a lifelong adventure that doesn't stop when you hit a specific weight target. It involves implementing long-term, sustainable lifestyle adjustments that improve your general well-being. This is a journey about learning to live a balanced existence in all areas of your life, not perfection.

Realize that the behaviors you've developed—mindful eating, consistent exercise, and stress-reduction methods—are the cornerstones of a better life rather than merely strategies for losing weight. These procedures ought to be established long-term rather than as band-aid solutions.

Continue to be inquisitive and receptive to learning about fitness, nutrition, and how your body reacts to this. Being informed gives you greater power, and the more informed you are, the more capable you will be of making decisions that promote your pleasure and well-being.

There will inevitably be setbacks, so be ready for them. Instead of seeing them as failures, though, see them as chances to become more determined. Remember that you have a daily opportunity to recommit to your health.

Keep up a network of friends, family, or community members who share your goals and values. They can support you, rejoice with you in your victories, and offer consolation when things are hard.

Finally, always remember to pay attention to your body and prioritize self-care. Take breaks when necessary, give your body what it needs, and partake in activities that feed your body and spirit.

You have a unique journey to wellness and health. It's an ongoing, dynamic process that develops and changes with you. It enhances your life in more ways than you may have thought if you really embrace it, with its ups and downs.

APPENDICES

DETAILED MEAL PLANS AND RECIPES FOR EACH BODY TYPE

You're about to explore extensive dietary advice specifically designed for each of the three basic body types—ectomorphs, mesomorphs, and endomorphs—in the appendix. Knowing your body type and its requirements is essential to designing a diet plan that works since every body type reacts differently to different foods and macronutrient ratios.

A. Overview of Body Types and Nutritional Requirements

Somatotypes, or body types, affect how you react to certain foods and exercise regimens. Usually, they fall into one of three categories:

1. The physiques of Ectomorphs are often long and thin. They may find it difficult to put on weight or muscle because of their quick metabolism. Because of their faster metabolic rates, ectomorphs frequently need more calories and may need to eat a higher percentage of carbs to stay energetic.

2. Mesomorphs frequently possess an innately athletic build and acquire muscle quite quickly. They may frequently more evenly balance their macronutrients and have a moderate metabolism. Their strong physique and busy lifestyle can be supported by a combination of proteins, lipids, and carbohydrates.

3. Endomorphs can put on weight quickly and typically have a rounder, more robust physique. They may benefit from a diet higher in fats and proteins and lower in carbohydrates because they frequently have slower metabolisms, which can aid with weight management and satiety.

While knowing your body type might help you make better dietary choices, there is no one-size-fits-all solution. There will always be differences between people. Therefore, it's important to consider additional elements like age, activity level, and personal objectives.

B. Utilizing the Recipes and Meal Plans

This appendix's meal plans and recipes are organized to meet the basic dietary requirements of every body type. Here's how to make good use of them:

1. Determine your body type to know where to begin creating your customized nutrition plan.
2. Modify the serving sizes according to your personal calorie requirements and objectives. You could need to eat fewer calories if you're trying to lose weight, but you might need to eat more to grow muscle.
3. Use the recipes as a guide; feel free to modify the ingredients according to availability, taste, or the time of year.
4. Organize your meals in advance to make sure you have everything you need and to prevent making rash food choices.
5. To help control your metabolism, Be consistent with the times you eat and make an effort to eat at roughly the same times every day.

C. Tailoring Recipes to Dietary Restrictions and Allergies

We are aware that dietary requirements can be complicated, particularly when taking into account dietary restrictions or allergies. You can alter these recipes as follows:

1. Allergy relief: Replace any allergens with appropriate substitutes. For instance, utilize sunflower or pumpkin seeds if you're allergic to nuts.
2. For intolerances: Choose lactose-free dairy or plant-based milk and cheese substitutes if you're intolerant to lactose.
3. For vegan or vegetarian diets: Use plant-based proteins such as tempeh, beans, lentils, or tofu instead of animal proteins. To increase your intake, plant-based protein powders are also available.
4. For those with gluten sensitivity: Swap out wheat-based items with gluten-free grains like rice, buckwheat, or quinoa.

When making big nutritional changes, always get advice from a doctor or nutritionist, particularly if you have any unique dietary requirements or medical issues. You can securely and successfully modify these designs with their assistance.

II. Recipes and Meal Plans for Ectomorphs

A. Overview of Ectomorph

Ectomorphs have a high metabolism and a slender physique, which makes it difficult for them to put on muscular mass. More calories are frequently required for them to experience bodily changes.

1. Needs for Macronutrients and Calories: Generally, ectomorphs need more calories than other body types to build bulk. Carbs should make up most of their macronutrient split; proteins should come in second for muscle repair and healthy fats for hormone regulation. A 50–60% carbohydrate, 25–30% protein, and 20–25% fat ratio could be optimal.

2. Value of Regular, High-Calorie Meals: Ectomorphs benefit from

eating more frequently—roughly every two to three hours—due to their quick metabolism. This can entail eating three main meals and significant snacks between them to maintain a high-calorie intake all day.

B. Ectomorphs' Weekly Meal Plan

To satisfy their increased energy needs, ectomorphs should follow a balanced diet that emphasizes foods high in nutrients and calories.

1. Breakfast, Lunch, Dinner, and Snacks from Day 1 to Day 7. -
   Breakfast: To start the day with energy, try something like avocado and egg toast or peanut butter banana oatmeal, which offer a combination of carbohydrates, protein, and healthy fats.
   - Buffet: Meals with a balanced protein and slow-releasing carbohydrates, such as bean salad and quinoa, are ideal for a midday energy boost.
   - Dinner: Recipes like creamy chicken Alfredo pasta offer a high-calorie, high-protein evening meal that helps repair muscles overnight.
   - Handsomes: To keep calorie intake in check during the day, try high-calorie protein smoothies or nutty granola bars between meals.

C. Cookbooks

The following dishes are made to be both nutrient-dense and high in energy to meet the high-calorie requirements of ectomorphs.

1. High Protein Shake Calorie:
   Blend together oats, peanut butter, banana, whey protein, and whole milk or a nondairy milk substitute. Drizzle with honey for additional carbohydrates.

2. Bean Salad with Quinoa:
   For a light and satisfying lunch, toss cooked quinoa with black

beans, sliced bell peppers, corn, cilantro, and lime vinaigrette.

3. Toasted Egg and Avocado:
Place poached eggs and mashed avocado on top of whole-grain bread. For a filling breakfast, add some salt and chili flakes.

4. Nut-filled Granola Bars:
Bake the oats, honey, mixed nuts, seeds, and dried fruits until they become crispy. These bars are ideal for eating on the run.

5. Banana Oatmeal with Peanut Butter:
For a creamy and filling breakfast, cook oats in your preferred milk and stir in banana slices and a liberal dollop of peanut butter.

6. Stuffed Avocados with Tuna Salad:
Combine mayonnaise, lemon juice, and any chosen herbs with canned tuna. Fill half of an avocado to make a high-protein, high-fat snack.

7. Creamy Alfredo Pasta with Chicken:
For a tasty, high-protein, and calorie-dense supper, sauté chicken breast and combine it with cooked fettuccine, cream, parmesan, and a dash of garlic.

Ectomorphs can use this meal plan and the foods that go with it as a model to boost muscular gain and fuel their rapid metabolisms. Ectomorphs must ensure they get enough calories and nutrients to support their daily activities and exercise, which will help them grow muscle and maintain a healthy weight.

III. Mesomorph Recipes and Meal Plans

A. Overview of Mesomorphs

Known for their athletic build, mesomorphs can acquire muscle and burn fat more easily than people with other body types. Their active lifestyle and body composition objectives are supported by a balanced distribution of macronutrients.

1. Achieving Macronutrient Balance for Gaining Muscle and Losing Fat: Carbs, proteins, and fats should be well-balanced in the diet of a mesomorph. Proteins are necessary for muscle growth and repair, while lipids sustain hormone balance and provide energy. Carbohydrates fuel strenuous exercise. For a mesomorph, a balanced macronutrient ratio might be 30% proteins, 40% carbohydrates, and 30% lipids.

2. The Significance of Meal Frequency and Timing: Mesomorphs usually manage three big meals plus a few snacks over the day. This frequency gives them a consistent supply of nutrients for muscular growth and recuperation, as well as assists their metabolism. It's important to time your meals, especially if you work out. Eating a mix of carbohydrates and protein before and after can help you recuperate and fuel your exercise.

B. Mesomorphs' Weekly Meal Plan

This meal plan emphasizes nutrient-dense, well-balanced meals to enhance a mesomorph's metabolism and ability to gain muscle.

1. Breakfast, Lunch, Dinner, and Snacks from Day 1 to Day 7. - Breakfast: Start the day with a balanced combination of macros with options like sweet potato and black bean bowls or Greek yogurt parfaits.

- Buffet: A substantial noon dosage of protein and fiber can be obtained from dishes like grilled chicken with avocado salad or turkey and quinoa stuffed peppers.

- Dinner: Full of protein and vital nutrients, dishes like stir-fried beef and broccoli or seared salmon with steamed vegetables provide a filling way to end the day.

- Handsomes: You may sustain energy and fullness between meals by having snacks like roasted chickpeas or a piece of fruit with a handful of nuts throughout the day.

C. Cookbooks

The balanced nutrition in these meals meets the needs of a mesomorph for both muscle growth and maintenance.

1. Greek Yogurt Parfait: To make a parfait that provides an excellent combination of protein, carbohydrates, and fats, layer Greek yogurt with granola, mixed berries, and honey.

2. Stuffed Peppers with Quinoa and Turkey:
   Bake bell peppers until softened after stuffing them with a mixture of cooked quinoa, diced tomatoes, ground turkey, and spices.

3. Avocado and Grilled Chicken Salad:
   For a light and satisfying salad, toss grilled chicken slices, avocado, mixed greens, cherry tomatoes, and a lemon-olive oil dressing.

Fourth, Roasted Chickpeas:
   For a high-protein and high-fiber snack, toss chickpeas with olive oil, cumin, paprika, and garlic powder and roast until crispy.

5. Brown Bean and Sweet Potato Bowl:
   For a well-balanced and delectable dinner, top a bowl of chopped roasted sweet potatoes and black beans with avocado, cheese, and salsa.

6. Steamed vegetables and seared salmon:
   Sear a fillet of salmon and serve it with steamed carrots and broccoli seasoned with lemon and herbs.

7. Beef and Broccoli Stir-Fry: For a high-protein supper, stir-fry beef and broccoli slices in a flavorful sauce over brown rice or quinoa.

Mesomorphs may encourage lean muscle growth and

maintenance while still getting the nutrition they need from these meal plans and recipes, which will fuel their exercises and aid in optimal recovery. Mesomorphs who adhere to these principles can better control their energy levels and body composition, making the most of their inherent advantages to reach their fitness objectives.

IV. Recipes and Meal Plans for Endomorphs

A. Overview of Endomorphs

Endomorphs frequently have rounder bodies and, because of their slower metabolism, can put on weight more quickly. A diet higher in proteins and fats and lower in carbohydrates may benefit them as it can aid in weight management.

1. High-Protein, Low-Carb, and Fat Loss Strategies: Endomorphs may consider eating a diet high in protein and good fats and low in carbohydrates, especially processed carbohydrates, to promote fat loss. This strategy lessens the chance of overeating by promoting a fullness sensation and helping to control insulin levels.

2. The Importance of Nutrient Density and Portion Control: Endomorphs must concentrate on portion management to limit their calorie consumption. The selected foods should be low in calories and nutrients, such as vitamins, minerals, and other elements that support general health.

B. Endomorph Weekly Meal Plan

This meal plan is designed with endomorphs' weight management objectives, emphasizing foods high in protein, low in carbohydrates, and healthy fats.

1. Breakfast, Lunch, Dinner, and Snacks from Day 1 to Day 7. - Breakfast: Low-carb options with lots of protein, such as egg muffins with spinach and mushrooms, are a great way to start the day.

- Buffet: Low-carb yet satisfying meals like stir-fried cauliflower rice are ideal for noon energy.

- Dinner: Light yet filling dishes such as grilled tilapia with lemon and herbs provide lean protein.

- Handsomes: Snacks like chicken lettuce wraps, or protein balls with almond and coconut can be utilized to sustain energy and fullness in between meals throughout the day.

C. Cookbooks

These dishes are made to offer a well-balanced diet appropriate for the nutritional requirements of an endomorph.

1. Mushroom and Spinach Egg Muffins:

Beat eggs, diced mushrooms, chopped spinach, and a small amount of cheese together. For a portable, high-protein breakfast, pour into muffin pans and bake until set.

2. Stir-fried cauliflower rice:

Add some veggies, such as bell peppers and snap peas, to riced cauliflower and sauté it. You may also add some protein, like tofu or shrimp. Add ginger and soy sauce for seasoning, and enjoy a tasty, low-carb supper.

3. Lemon and Herb Broiled Tilapia:

Tilapia fillets are seasoned with olive oil, thyme, and lemon zest. Serve the flaky fish with steamed greens, such as zucchini or asparagus, and broil it for a few minutes.

4. Protein Balls with Almond and Coconut Flour:

Add shredded coconut, protein powder, almond butter, and a drizzle of honey. Form into balls and store in the fridge until solid for an easy, high-protein snack.

5. Avocado and Kale Smoothie:

Blended kale leaves, half an avocado, unsweetened almond milk, and a scoop of protein powder make this smoothie rich in healthy fats and protein.

6. Wrapped Lettuce Chicken:
   Cook ground chicken in a flavorful sauce with onions and garlic. Serve in lettuce leaves for a pleasant, low-carb, light supper.

7. Pesto Chicken over Zucchini Noodles:
   Noodles made from spiralized zucchini are combined with grilled chicken strips and homemade pesto. This meal is a great option for dinner because it's robust in taste and low in carbohydrates.

Endomorphs can control how many macronutrients they eat to aid in weight loss by implementing these dishes into their meal plans. A balanced diet and the maintenance of a healthy metabolism will depend on portion control, meal planning, and the selection of nutrient-dense foods. Endomorphs can cooperate with their body type to preserve health and wellness if they put these tactics in place.

V. Extras and Snacks

A well-planned snack can help control hunger, give you energy between meals, and increase your consumption of nutrients overall. Snacks should be carefully selected to fulfill the unique requirements of your body type and to balance off your main meals of the day.

A. Nutritious Snacks for Every Body Style

1. Mixed Nuts and Seeds: A little portion of mixed nuts and seeds offers a healthy ratio of fiber, lipids, and proteins, making it a nutrient-dense snack. Good options include almonds, walnuts, pumpkin seeds, and sunflower seeds. They provide protein, important fatty acids, and other micronutrients that help with satiety, brain function, and muscle regeneration.

2. Greek Yogurt with Berries: Packed with gut-friendly bacteria

and excellent protein, Greek yogurt is a great snack. Berries complement it with natural sweetness, fiber, and antioxidants. For mesomorphs, who need protein to maintain muscle, and ectomorphs, who frequently need more calories throughout the day, this combination can be especially helpful.

3. Cottage Cheese and Fruit: Cottage cheese is a great source of protein and makes a satisfying snack when combined with fruit like peaches or pineapple. The high protein and low sugar content will help endomorphs regulate their weight.

4. Vegetable Sticks with Hummus: High in fiber and low in calories are veggies, including bell peppers, carrots, and celery. Chickpea-based hummus provides good lipids and protein. With its excellent nutritional content and moderate calorie content, this snack is satisfying for endomorphs.

B. Dressings & Sauces

1. Homemade Vinaigrette: For a quick and healthful salad dressing, combine olive oil, vinegar, mustard, and herbs. Olive oil's beneficial lipids can aid in absorbing fat-soluble vitamins from your vegetables.

2. Greek Tzatziki Sauce: To make a cool, creamy sauce, mix Greek yogurt with grated cucumber, garlic, lemon juice, and dill. Because of its high protein content and good fats, it works well as a condiment for grilled meats or vegetable dip and is suitable for all body types.

3. Spicy Avocado Dressing: For a creamy dressing with a bite, blend one avocado with lime juice, cilantro, garlic, and jalapeño. This is a fantastic method to supplement your meal with good fats, which will help you feel fuller for longer.

4. Tomato and Basil Marinara: To create a nutrient-rich sauce that pairs well with grilled chicken or zucchini noodles, simmer

crushed tomatoes with basil, garlic, onion, and olive oil.

C. Shakes and Smoothies

1. Chocolate Peanut Butter Protein Shake: Blend peanut butter, banana, and your preferred milk with a scoop of chocolate protein powder. Ectomorphs that need an extra burst of protein and calories should try this smoothie.

2. Antioxidant Berry Smoothie: For a nutrient-dense beverage, blend almond milk, spinach, mixed berries, and a scoop of protein powder. All body types benefit from the antioxidants in berries, which promote general health.

3. Green Detox Smoothie: Combine kale or spinach with cucumber, lemon juice, green apple, and ginger for a revitalizing beverage. An endomorph's diet plan can benefit greatly from including this low-calorie smoothie.

4. Vanilla Almond Protein Shake: For a quick and filling shake, blend almond milk, almond butter, and vanilla protein powder with ice. It can be made into a satisfying snack or meal replacement by adding a spoonful of chia seeds to boost the fiber content.

Whether you're searching for a satisfying drink, a tasty supplement to your meals, or a quick snack, these products meet various dietary requirements and may be tailored to meet your personal fitness and health objectives. To maintain a healthy and balanced diet, remember to factor in these extras in your total meal plan.

VI. Final Thoughts

Achieving and sustaining your fitness and health goals can be achieved by transforming your lifestyle with an organized food plan and recipe book. When you wrap up this extensive book, consider these strategies to guarantee longevity and flexibility in your dietary path.

A. Advice on Preparing and Storing Meals

One very useful tactic to help you stick to your diet plan is meal prep. It helps avoid bad eating decisions, saves time, and lowers stress. The following advice will help you prepare meals more effectively:

1. Plan Ahead: Make a meal and snack plan for the coming week before it starts. This foresight stops you from making rash judgments that might not align with your objectives.

2. Shop Smart: Make a list of everything you need to buy based on your meal plan to reduce waste and save money.

3. Batch Cook: At the start of the week, make big servings of adaptable foods like grains, veggies, and proteins. Mix and combine these to make various meals that keep your diet fresh.

4. Appropriate Storage: Make an investment in high-quality, BPA-free, microwave-safe containers. To maintain freshness, portion your meals and mark them with the date.

5. Freeze for Longevity: You can freeze some meals and thaw them later to make sure you always have a wholesome choice available. Freezing soups, stews, and casseroles is a terrific idea.

6. Prep Snacks: To avoid overindulging and to make it convenient to grab a snack on the run, portion up snacks into separate servings.

B. Modifying Meal Schedules to Meet Changing Fitness Objectives

As your exercise objectives change, so will your nutritional requirements. You must modify your eating plan to accommodate these adjustments:

1. Increased exercise: You might require extra calories if your level of exercise rises. Include high-calorie snacks or bigger meal portions to satisfy your energy needs.

2. Muscle Gain: To enhance muscle growth and repair, prioritize protein consumption. Consider enhancing your meals with extra lean protein sources or a protein supplement.

3. Fat Loss: If cutting fat is the main objective, concentrate on establishing a calorie deficit by controlling portion sizes and giving lower-calorie, nutrient-dense foods priority.

4. Endurance Training: To replace glycogen stores, endurance athletes would require a higher carbohydrate intake. For a healthier diet, consider including complex carbohydrates like quinoa, brown rice, and sweet potatoes.

5. Regular Review: Check that your meal plan aligns with your current fitness objectives every few weeks and make any required adjustments.

C. Motivation to Persist in Investigating Individual Nutrition

Lastly, see your journey toward a healthy diet as a continuous educational process. Your understanding of your body's demands and your relationship with food will continue to change. Remember these guidelines as you proceed:

1. Listen to Your Body: Observe your body's reactions to various foods. You can choose the healthiest foods by paying attention to how your body responds.

2. Remain Up to Date: Nutrition research is constantly progressing. Keep up with the latest findings and think about how they can relate to your situation.

3. Seek Professional Advice: If you have specific health problems or

are making major dietary changes, don't hesitate to speak with a dietitian or nutritionist.

4. Experiment: Try different foods and recipes without fear. Variety helps guarantee a wide intake of nutrients and keep your diet interesting.

5. Pardon Mistakes: Everyone indulges occasionally. You must go back to your strategy guilt-free and without any hesitation.

6. Celebrate Successes: Regardless of how little your accomplishments may have been, give them some thought. Rewarding yourself for your accomplishments is essential to staying motivated.

Recall that nutritious food is essential to living a vigorous and fulfilling life, not merely as fuel. You may prime yourself for a lifetime of well-being by cooking nourishing and satisfying meals, adjusting to your plan, and keeping up your nutrition education. Continue investigating, adjusting, and relishing the trip toward optimal well-being.

WORKOUT TEMPLATES AND EXERCISE DEMONSTRATIONS

Exercise Examples and Workout Templates

Customizing your workout to meet your unique objectives, tastes, and lifestyle is a dynamic process that necessitates a basic knowledge of workout design and effective exercise performance. You may guarantee that your workouts are efficient, safe, and effective by using workout templates and paying attention to exercise demonstrations.

Fitness Routines

An exercise schedule template acts as a guide for organizing your workouts. Focusing on all the main muscle groups and combining various training modalities like strength, cardio, and flexibility guarantees a well-rounded approach.

1. Complete-Body Power Model:

   - Warm-up: 5–10 minutes of dynamic stretching and mild aerobic

   - Upper Body: Pull exercises (like rows) and Push exercises (like push-ups)

   - Lower Body: Squat exercises (such as goblet squats) and Hinge exercises (such as deadlifts)

   - Core: Stabilization (like planks) and Rotation (like Russian twists)

- Cool-down: Static stretching for five to ten minutes

2. Template for Cardio Circuit:
- Warm-up: vigorous walking or jogging for five to ten minutes
The circuit: Repeat three to four sets of two to three minutes of intense exercise (burpees, jumping jacks, high knees, etc.), followed by one minute of rest or low-intensity activity.
- Cool-down: 5–10 minutes of static stretching and a gradually reduced level of activity

3. Template for Flexibility and Mobility:
- Light aerobics for five minutes to warm up
- Dynamic stretching: arm circles, torso twists, and leg swings
- Static stretching: Focus on the main muscle groups by holding each stretch for 15 to 30 seconds.
- Mobility exercises: ankle, shoulder, and hip rolls

Demonstrations of Exercise
It's essential to comprehend the right form and technique to perform exercises safely and correctly. Exercise demonstrations give you verbal and visual cues to help you with each movement, whether following along with a trainer or watching tutorial videos.

1. Strength Training: - Exercises such as bench presses and squats should all have examples showing the beginning posture, movement phase, breathing technique, and return to the starting position. To prevent harm, pay close attention to the typical errors indicated in the demonstrations.

2. Cardio Exercises: - Exercises like burpees and mountain climbers will be demonstrated, emphasizing the value of keeping a steady rhythm and correct technique even when exhaustion sets in. To ensure efficacy and safety, regulated motions should take precedence over speed.

3. Mobility and Flexibility: - Stretching demonstrations should highlight appropriate alignment and how to gradually get into

each position to prevent overstretching. Mobility exercises will frequently show you how to go through a range of motion and execute each motion smoothly and slowly.

Including Templates and Examples in Your Daily Activities
To include these in your daily routine:
1. Select the Correct Template: Make sure the exercise plan you choose aligns with your objectives. Choose the full-body strength template if your goal is to gain strength. Choose the cardio circuit if your goal is to improve your cardiovascular health.

2. Learn the Exercises: To ensure that you perform new exercises correctly, view demos or speak with an expert before incorporating them into your program.

3. Customize Your Workouts: Start with the templates and adjust them to meet your fitness level, the availability of the equipment, and your own tastes.

4. Track Your Progress: Record the exercises, weights, repetitions, and sets you do in your workout journal. This will enable you to track your development and make the required corrections.

5. Maintain Consistency: It takes consistency to get forward. To give your body time to adjust, follow your selected template for a few weeks before making any alterations.

You can design an organized, diverse, and safe exercise program to help you get closer to your fitness objectives by using workout templates and paying attention to exercise demonstrations. Recall that achieving fitness is a unique and dynamic journey. As you make progress, have patience, and don't be afraid to ask for help when you need it.

RESOURCES FOR FURTHER READING AND SUPPORT

Access to high-quality resources before starting a health and fitness journey can provide the information and encouragement you need to reach your objectives. The following resources can be very helpful for anyone looking to learn more and find support:

1. Books:
   - **Anti-Inflammatory Diet Meal Prep** by Ginger Hultin
   - **Eat What You Love, Love What You Eat** by Michelle May
   - **Embrace You: Your Guide to Transforming Weight Loss Misconceptions Into Lifelong Wellness** by Sylvia Gonsahn-Bollie
   - **Embody: Learning to Love Your Unique Body** by Connie Sobczak
   - **Fierce Self-Compassion** by Kristin Neff.

2. Websites:
   - **The Mediterranean Diet** - Website
   - **Noom** - Website
   - **Nutrisystem** - Website
   - **The New Mayo Clinic Diet**
   - **Whole30** - Website
   - **WW (WeightWatchers)** - Website

3. Apps:
   - **Calorie Counter** by MyNetDiary

- **Calorie Counter by FatSecret**
- **Calorie Counter** by Lose It!
- **Fitbit**
- **MyFitnessPal** by Calorie Counter

Podcasts:
- **Free Method Podcast**
- **Gluten Free Weigh In**
- **The Cabral Concept**
- **The Exam Room by the Physicians Committee**
- **You Won't Believe What I Ate Last Night**

These resources can provide the extra information and inspiration you need to keep moving forward with your journey toward health and wellness. Recall that community support and ongoing education are essential elements of long-lasting change.

www.ingramcontent.com/pod-product-compliance
Lightning Source LLC
Chambersburg PA
CBHW070947260726
48661CB00003B/1169